Lesser Harms

MORALITY AND SOCIETY SERIES

Edited by Alan Wolfe

LESSER HARMS

The Morality of Risk in Medical Research

SYDNEY A. HALPERN

The University of Chicago Press
Chicago and London

Sydney A. Halpern is professor of sociology and medical humanities at the University of Illinois at Chicago. She is author of *American Pediatrics: The Social Dynamics of Professionalism, 1880–1920.*

The University of Chicago Press, Chicago 60637
The University of Chicago Press, Ltd., London
© 2004 by The University of Chicago
All rights reserved. Published 2004
Printed in the United States of America
13 12 11 10 09 08 07 06 05 04   5 4 3 2 1

ISBN (cloth): 0-226-31451-0

Library of Congress Cataloging-in-Publication Data

Halpern, Sydney A. (Sydney Ann)
    Lesser harms : the morality of risk in medical research / Sydney A. Halpern.
        p.   cm. — (Morality and society series)
    Includes bibliographical references and index.
    ISBN 0-226-31451-0 (cloth : alk. paper)
    1. Human experimentation in medicine—Moral and ethical aspects—United States.
    2. Medicine—Research—Moral and ethical aspects—United States.   3. Medicine—
    Research—Law and legislation—United States.   4. Poliomyelitis vaccine—Research—
    Moral and ethical aspects—United States.   I. Title.   II. Morality and society.
    R853.H8H357   2004
    174.2′8—dc22

                                                                2004002322

⊚ The paper used in this publication meets the minimum requirements of the American National Standard for Information Sciences—Permanence of Paper for Printed Library Materials, ANSI Z39.48-1992.

In memory of Phyllis E. Halpern

Contents

Acknowledgments

Archivists and records managers were indispensable to the collection of documentary materials on which this book is based. I am very grateful for the assistance of Beth Carroll-Horrocks and Martin Levitt at the American Philosophical Society; Lauren Lassleben at the Bancroft Library; Nancy Bartlett at the Bentley Historical Library; Billie Broaddus at the Cincinnati Medical Heritage Center; Kevin Crawford and Jack Eckert at the College of Physicians of Philadelphia; Elizabeth Denier at the Franklin D. Roosevelt Library; Geoffrey Wexler at the Mandeville Library; Bob Diorio and Robert Gelles at the March of Dimes; Marjorie Ciarlante, Wil Mahoney, and Aloha South at the National Archives; Richard Mandel and Dave Porter at the Office of the Director of the National Institutes of Health (NIH); Robert Jambou at the NIH Office of Biotechnology Activities; Gabriel Jervais and William Lovett at New York City's Bush Terminal repository; Lola Martin at the New York Foundation; Margaret Jerrido at Temple University's Urban Archives. Tom Rosenbaum at the Rockefeller Archive Center was exceptionally helpful in his extensive knowledge of collection and his generosity with his time.

While researching and writing the book, I received support from multiple sources. I undertook the initial examination of archival records with the help of travel-to-collection awards from the American Philosophical Society, the Bentley Historical Library of the University of Michigan, the College of Physicians of Philadelphia, the Humanities Institute of the University of Illinois at Chicago, the National Endowment for the Humanities (NEH),

and the Rockefeller Archive Center. The NEH provided additional funding
for the project through a summer stipend, a university fellowship, and a research grant from the NEH Program on Humanities, Science, and Technology. I am indebted to Daniel Jones, NEH program officer for the grant, for
making the project's administration seamless. Two units at the University
of Illinois at Chicago contributed to the book's completion: the Humanities
Institute, offering fellowship support and stimulating interaction with a diverse group of scholars, and the Institute for Government and Public Affairs
(IGPA), providing a visiting faculty position and collegiality during the final
stages of the manuscript's preparation. For these opportunities, I thank
Mary Beth Rose at the Humanities Institute and Jack Knott at IGPA. Several
other institutions also extended generous hospitality. During my tenure as
an NEH Fellow, David Rothman graciously arranged a courtesy appointment for me at Columbia University's Center of the Study of Society and
Medicine. Thanks also to Arthur Caplan and other faculty at the Center for
Bioethics at the University of Pennsylvania for welcoming me as a visiting
scholar during the summer and fall of 2000.

A number of people read and offered substantive responses to portions
of the book-in-progress. For their comments on one or more book chapters,
I owe a debt of gratitude to Charles Bosk, Robert Cook-Deegan, Joel Frader,
Andrew Jameton, Pamela Popielarz, Andrea Rusnock, and Janet Tighe.
Renée Anspach responded graciously to multiple versions of portions of the
manuscript. Joel Howell and Carol Heimer provided invaluable critiques of
the draft manuscript as a whole that were the basis for final revisions. I benefited also from the observations of a broader range of scholars who commented on presentations and conference papers related to the book. I received additional assistance from students at the University of Illinois at
Chicago, including Wei Hong, Nancy Maloney, Elise Martel, Kristin Nicode-
mus, and Alizah Rotramel.

I have already thanked privately the family and close friends whose emo-
tional support sustained me through the long haul of writing this book. But
my public acknowledgments would not be complete without an expression
of gratitude to Doug Mitchell at the University of Chicago Press for shep-
herding the manuscript through the publication process; to Alan Wolfe, series editor, for his enthusiasm from the start; and to my copyeditor, Carlisle
Rex-Waller, for her patience through my final adjustments to the book.

Abbreviations

AEB	Army Epidemiology Board
AFEB	Armed Forces Epidemiology Board
AMA	American Medical Association
APHA	American Public Health Association
BRMAC	Biological Response Modifiers Advisory Committee
CBER	Center for Biologics Evaluation and Research
CDER	Center for Drug Evaluation and Research
CMR	Committee on Medical Research
CRC	Clinical Research Committee
DCGT	Division of Cellular and Gene Therapy
DHHS	U.S. Department of Health and Human Services
DRL	Dermatological Research Institute
FDA	U.S. Food and Drug Administration
ICM	Institute of Cutaneous Medicine
IHD	International Health Division of the Rockefeller Foundation
IHGT	Institute for Human Gene Therapy
IND	investigational new drug
IRB	institutional review board
JAMA	*Journal of the American Medical Association*
LIMC	Long Island Medical College
NIH	National Institutes of Health (National Institute of Health between 1930 and 1944)
NSMR	National Society for Medical Research

NUCDF   National Urea Cycle Disorders Foundation
OHRP   Office for Human Research Protections
OSRD   Office of Scientific Research and Development
OTC   Ornithine transcarbamylase
PBBC   President's Birthday Ball Commission
RAC   Recombinant DNA Advisory Committee

Introduction

Many depictions of clinical research appearing in American publications during the final third of the twentieth century are strikingly incompatible with the notion of morality. In the 1960s and 1970s, the use of human subjects in medical research came under public and professional scrutiny. Critics insisted that scientists were routinely committing investigatory abuses: exposing subjects to undue risks, drawing subjects from vulnerable groups, and failing to obtain informed consent. Reports of research excesses flooded the popular press and triggered policy debate within Congress and federal agencies. The result was a system of regulatory oversight now familiar to virtually all clinical researchers and a great many social and behavioral scientists. In the early 1960s, the Food and Drug Administration issued new codes governing the experimental use of unlicensed medical products. Later that decade, the National Institutes of Health mandated peer review of human-subjects protocols by locally constituted institutional review boards. Federally sponsored commissions composed of scholars in the emerging field of bioethics convened during the 1970s and 1980s to refine the standards used in the evaluations of these local boards. Two imperatives were central to the newly articulated research ethics: freely given, informed consent and protection of subjects from unreasonable risks.[1]

Commentators have pointed to a number of developments that helped shape the new regulatory standards: the Nuremberg codes of the late 1940s, court rulings in the late 1950s that defined the meaning of informed consent, movements for patients' rights during the 1960s, and the consolidation of bioethics as a scholarly field and policy arena in the 1970s.[2] Some of the earliest advocates for change were academic physicians. Henry Beecher, a Harvard anesthesiologist, sharply criticized investigators' treatment of human subjects in a 1966 paper published in the *New England Journal of Medicine*.[3] But most observers have seen the impetus for research ethics as exogenous to medical science. The impression left by exposés of the 1960s and 1970s is that, in the absence of ethical codes and oversight procedures imposed from outside, researchers would apply few constraints upon their own or their colleagues' investigatory conduct.

Postwar indictments of abuses notwithstanding, a growing body of scholarship points to longstanding moral traditions among medical researchers—traditions quite distinct from those associated with bioethics as it emerged during the 1960s and 1970s.[4] The bioethical tenets institutionalized in regulatory codes are formally codified and based largely on ideas and principles—about autonomy, equity, and individual rights—originating from outside the profession of medicine. In contrast, the profession's moral traditions are informal, uncodified, and indigenous to communities of scientists. Researchers typically voice their traditions in a fragmentary manner and often find it difficult to disentangle professional morality from convictions about the theories and methods of science. Presented unsystematically and subject to shifting constructions, moral traditions have nonetheless powerfully influenced the conduct of clinical research for well over a century.

In this book, I examine moral traditions governing the introduction of new medical interventions before the advent of federal regulation and formal bioethics. My empirical focus is vaccine innovation in America during the early and middle decades of the twentieth century. I also touch on earlier vaccine controversies in Europe and, in later sections of the book, expand the discussion to a broader range of clinical research. My central purpose throughout is to clarify patterns in the management of hazards that inevitably accompany use of new medical procedures. I draw on data from an array of secondary and primary historical sources, including materials collected at more than a dozen archival repositories.

In elaborating moral traditions for testing risk-laden medical procedures, I am not suggesting that these alone are sufficient to prevent excesses by researchers. Even if the scope and content of scientists' indigenous morality were adequate to that task, having moral precepts and enacting them are two different matters. The latter—as this analysis shows—is considerably more difficult to accomplish. My goal is neither to applaud nor debunk. Rather, my hope is to clarify the character of moral traditions in medical science, patterns in their implementation, their evolution over time, and the ways that indigenous moralities have affected and continue to affect the conduct of human research.

Indigenous Morality among Clinical Researchers

The statements and practices of working scientists provide abundant evidence for moral traditions within clinical-research communities. No comprehensive picture of these traditions is available in existing literature. But a portrait can be constructed from primary sources and from the scholarship of historians and ethnographers who study medical scientists. One of the remarkable features of clinical investigators' morality is its longevity. Researchers' moral traditions precede by many decades the Nuremberg codes and the advent of bioethics. Susan Lederer has examined human experiments conducted in the United States during the first four decades of the twentieth century. She concludes that "at no time were American investigators free to do whatever they pleased with their human subjects. Neither their peers nor the public would have stood for reckless experimentation."[5] The content of researchers' indigenous morality is also remarkable. Concern with both consent and protection from harm—core issues in late-twentieth-century bioethics—has long been at the center of scientists' moral traditions. In 1907, the eminent late-nineteenth-century academic physician William Osler discussed the morality of medical research in an address to the Congress of American Physicians and Surgeons. He insisted that two conditions make human experiments allowable: "absolute safety" and "full consent." Osler immediately amended the stipulation of absolute safety, however, remarking that "risk to the individual may be taken with his consent and full knowledge."[6]

At the time of Osler's address, consent seeking was already an identifiable feature of the culture of medical practice. Historian Martin Pernick finds sensitivity to the issue of consent in both medical and legal case records and in statements by physicians that reveal an unexpected level of concern with the patient's role in medical decision making. Pernick argues that "truth-telling and consent seeking" were "part of an indigenous medical tradition" among American physicians as far back as the eighteenth century.[7] His account has triggered protests from members of the bioethics community, who object that etiquette among eighteenth-century physicians has little in common with today's consent practices.[8] But Pernick underscores that early views of consent differed in both content and purpose from modern notions. Ideas of consent in the present-day bioethics literature are grounded in the principle of autonomy, the patient's right to make decisions about his or her own treatment. Indigenous consent practices are based on the notion of beneficence, the doctor's duty to take action that is in the patient's interest. If eighteenth-century physicians thought it advisable to tell patients the truth and to seek their consent, it was because contemporary medical theories taught that, in many cases, knowledge had a beneficial effect on patients' health.

Beneficence has also influenced physicians' approach to consent when their interventions have been deliberate experiments. Among early-twentieth-century medical researchers, rules for consent were contingent on both the status of the subject and the expected outcome of the intervention. Clinical investigators considered experiments with healthy subjects to be different from those with patients. They also drew distinctions between therapeutic and nontherapeutic interventions. Physicians were obliged to obtain consent when experimenting on healthy subjects. They were also obliged to inform subjects and obtain consent when experimentation involved "discomfort and risk . . . without the promise of therapeutic benefit."[9] But when the subject was a patient and the medical procedure was expected to yield therapeutic benefit, physician beneficence ruled and researchers did not consider consent to be mandatory.

Primary and secondary literatures not only attest to a long history of consent practices, they also reveal well-established traditions for addressing the hazards that accompany clinical experiments. A core tradition for handling risk is the logic of lesser harms. According to this logic, use of an intervention is justified if the risks it entails are lower than the risks of the natural disease that the intervention is designed to prevent or treat. Pernick dates lesser-harm reasoning to the mid-nineteenth century and links its appearance to the growing influence of science on the culture of medicine. He suggests that lesser-harm reasoning drew on work, particularly that of Pierre Louis, conducted at the Paris Hospital during the 1830s.[10] Louis advocated the systematic evaluation of medical therapies using empirical observation, experimental controls, and statistical comparisons. Many physicians resisted applying empirical methods to clinical therapies, but scientific approaches nonetheless importantly influenced medical practice in both Europe and America. Pernick notes that medical thought in nineteenth-century America was divided over the preferability of letting disease run its natural course or engaging in heroic intervention. A new resolution emerged at midcentury to select a course of action that minimized overall harm from both illness and medical treatment. American physicians applied this logic when introducing anesthesia into medical practice in the

1850s. They collected and published numerical evidence comparing surgical mortality rates with and without anesthetics in an effort to determine whether the net impact of anesthetics was "beneficial or prejudicial."[11]

Today, lesser-harm reasoning is widespread both in medical research and clinical practice. Sociologists Renée Fox and Judith Swazey asked state-of-the-art transplantation surgeons how they decide when to use a new surgical procedure. Their respondents answered without hesitation: "One weighs the mortality of the disease against the mortality of the operation." If the patient's condition is terminal, surgery that appreciably raises chances for survival is justified, even if the intervention is very risky. But if the patient's condition is not life threatening, even a tiny surgical death rate is unacceptable.[12] Lesser-harm reasoning is by no means limited to surgeons. Medical practitioners and researchers of all types weigh the mortality and complication rates of new interventions against those of standard medical treatments and untreated disease. The probabilistic character of this reasoning has earned it the label "statistical morality."[13]

When applying lesser-harm reasoning in clinical practice, physicians focus on risks and benefits to the individual being treated. When considering research to test a medical innovation, investigators consider the anticipated outcomes not only for the experiment's subjects but also for medical knowledge and future patients. The tradition involves a utilitarian calculus. Lesser-harm logic requires the probability of net benefit. But risk to subjects can be balanced by the expectation of a contribution to the greater social good.

While lesser-harm reasoning spans medical practice and medical science, four additional traditions for handling risk are specific to research. The first links moral assessments to the theories and methods of empirical science. Investigators insist that only technically sound experiments are moral because scientifically invalid studies cannot advance medical knowledge or contribute to the collective good. Harry Marks notes the importance of scientific criteria in researchers' moral judgments when examining debates among American scientists in 1942–43 about risk-laden experiments designed to test treatments for gonorrhea. Marks concludes that there was a well-established, if not thoroughly articulated morality within the medical-research community, one that linked scientific principles with moral ones.[14] David Rutstein, an academic physician who conducted clinical tests of streptomycin during the 1940s, put his take on this matter succinctly: "The scientific validity of a study on human beings is in itself an ethical principle." He continues: "a poorly or improperly designed study" that is unable to yield scientific facts "cannot possibly benefit anyone. Any risk to the patient, however small, cannot be justified."[15]

Second, researchers have been committed to testing medical innovations on animals before introducing them in clinical practice. "The final test
of every new procedure, medical or surgical must be made on man," Osler
declared, "but never before it is first tried on animals."[16] Present-day researchers also cite animal testing as a moral prerequisite for human experiments. As one physician-innovator put it, "laboratory study puts the stamp
of human and ethical acceptability on therapeutic innovation more than any
other characteristic."[17] Animal experiments are crucial in part because they
provide a basis for initial assessments of safety and efficacy. It is from laboratory studies that researchers make estimates of the risks and benefits of
clinical innovations when data from human trials are not yet available.

A third accompaniment of lesser-harm reasoning is the expectation that
researchers will delay or suspend human applications of an intervention if
the hazards of a procedure are too grave. Fox and Swazey, who first identified
these hiatuses, call them "clinical moratoria." When a moratorium is ongoing, researchers limit their experiments to laboratory studies and endeavor
to lower risks before resuming human testing. Observers of recent developments in clinical research have described moratoria in the human use of
mitral-valve surgery, artificial heart implants, heart transplantation, other
transplant procedures, and recombinant DNA therapy.[18]

A final tradition for handling investigatory hazards is the practice of self-
experimentation. Here, researchers try risk-laden interventions on themselves before embarking on tests with a broader range of human subjects.
In his 1986 study of self-experimentation, Lawrence Altman provides examples of the practice from a wide range of clinical-research fields. Self-
experimentation attests to the investigator's confidence in the safety of an
innovation and demonstrates the willingness to place his or her own well-
being at risk before asking others to do so.[19] As Lederer remarks, the practice has undeniable public relations value. Professional leaders have lauded
self-experimentation when defending human research. Osler's comments
on the subject are illustrative. "The history of our profession," he writes, "is
starred with the heroism of its members who have sacrificed health and
sometimes life itself in endeavors to benefit their fellow creatures."[20]

The Inconsistent Application of Moral Traditions

Primary and secondary literatures provide the basis for a comprehensive
picture of moral traditions among medical researchers. These traditions include attention to both the consent of subjects and their protection from undue hazards. But a persistent duality emerges from historical and ethno-

graphic sources. While the empirical record attests to longstanding informal traditions, it also reveals tremendous inconsistency in whether and how they are implemented. Scholars familiar with clinical experimentation during the early and middle decades of the twentieth century could cite numerous instances where researchers have failed to observe the prevailing morality. Indigenous traditions exist, but how clinical researchers implement them is highly variable.

For example, erratic use of consent procedures generated comment from the authors of the 1995 report of the Advisory Committee on Human Radiation Experiments. They note "a strong tradition of consent . . . in research with healthy subjects" during the 1940s and 1950s, particularly where experiments "offered no prospect of medical benefit to the participant." Yet researchers who were certainly familiar with contemporary norms "sometimes employed unconsenting healthy subjects in research that offered them no medical benefit."[21] Early- and midcentury clinical investigators were also inconsistent in their use of procedures for managing risk. Although some researchers engaged in self-experimentation, many others did not. Animal testing was more nearly universal, at least among innovators who considered their interventions to be experiments. Where feasible, many clinical investigators tested new procedures with animals prior to human trials. But researchers differed considerably in the extent to which they required problems accompanying clinical innovations to be solved in the laboratory before trying new therapies on humans. And interpretations of lesser-harm logic varied greatly. In some cases, researchers scrupulously refrained from initiating human use of incompletely tested or very hazardous procedures. In others—as exposés published in the 1960s remind us—investigators proceeded with risk-laden interventions offering little or no benefit to human subjects.

If, as I assert, researchers' informal norms are longstanding and widespread, then what accounts for marked variation in the application of moral traditions? I return to this question numerous times in this book. For the moment, several observations about the traditions themselves serve as my starting point. While scientists' informal morality is enduring and pervasive, numerous ambiguities are embedded within the traditions and researchers encounter many quandaries in the course of applying them.[22] For example, norms governing consent have prescribed different actions depending on whether the intervention is a therapeutic procedure or a deliberate experiment. But the line separating therapy and research is often blurred. Fox and Swazey argue that no clear dichotomy exists. They propose an experiment-therapy continuum whereby newly introduced medical interventions proceed in increments to assume the status of being standard treatments.[23] Furthermore, many clinicians have had little hesitation in using untested therapeutic procedures as measures of last resort in the treatment of terminally ill patients. In such cases, physicians have considered their interventions to be therapeutic procedures rather than experiments. Defined this way, neither full disclosure of risks nor preliminary animal trials were considered mandatory.

Quandaries surrounding the application of lesser-harm reasoning are no less tricky. Researchers encounter at least two types of indeterminacy when trying to balance the potential risks and benefits of a new therapy against the dangers of natural disease. First, the terms of lesser-harm logic are inherently ambiguous. Researchers' indigenous morality does not indicate what ratio of benefits to hazards makes an intervention acceptable. Nor does it specify precisely what outcomes to consider when making risk-benefit calculations. Should researchers limit their calculations to mortality rates or should other consequences of natural disease and experimental interventions be considered as well? How should these different outcomes be weighed? Are patients' perceptions of risks and benefits to be factored in? When evaluating the benefits of a human experiment, should scientists place priority on outcomes for future patients and society at large or for the subjects participating in that particular experiment?[24] Scientists' informal morality provides little clear guidance on these issues, which have been the focal point of recurrent controversy among clinical investigators.

A second source of indeterminacy in applying lesser-harm reasoning arises from the uncertainties of interpreting scientific evidence.[25] I noted earlier that researchers base their judgments about an experiment's benefits at least in part on their assessment of its scientific validity. Moral judgments are contingent on scientific ones in another way as well. Researchers' estimates of an experiment's risks and benefits rest also on their interpretation of existing empirical evidence. But such evidence is open to multiple interpretations, and researchers often disagree in their assessments. The meaning of empirical findings is the subject of continual debate and negotiation among scientists. Social processes are crucial to the conduct and outcome of such negotiations.[26]

These observations point to a vitally important source of variation in scientists' application of indigenous moralities. Researchers are inconsistent in implementing their moral traditions because a variety of social dynamics influence their judgments and actions. Some of these dynamics concern the evaluation of empirical evidence and assessments of scientific validity. Some involve the framing, construction, and weighing of experimental risks and benefits. Some concern incentives and constraints created by the sponsors of human experiments, the legal system, the contemporary cultural climate, and scientists' relations with the broader public.

The Social Character of Moral Action

In this volume, I examine the social processes that have shaped the emergence and expression of researchers' indigenous moralities. I am not the first to suggest that social contingencies affect investigatory morality in medicine. Writing in the 1970s, sociologist Bernard Barber addressed the impact of social-structural factors on the moral inclinations of individual researchers. Barber's group questioned a sample of clinical investigators about their interpretation of informed consent and their willingness to pursue risk-laden protocols. The group concluded that whether a researcher is strict or permissive in moral orientation rests on his or her level of productivity and position within the reward structure of science.[27] While I also emphasize the impact of social factors, my focus is not the moral stances of individual researchers but rather the collective judgments of scientific communities. Individual conscience does, without doubt, affect scientists' willingness to embark upon or refrain from risky experiments. But individuals are rarely unilateral moral actors. They are embedded in communities that frame moral issues, designate which issues matter, and provide repertoires for managing moral problems. Furthermore, scientists routinely make collective judgments as to whether risky experiments are justifiable.

Collective deliberations about the acceptability of research hazards take place at a number of different sites. In America today, locally constituted institutional review boards assess human-subjects protocols. Federal agencies issue standards to govern board evaluations, and national bioethics commissions, convened periodically since the 1960s, codify the bases for these regulations. But two social units have long been central in formulating and implementing moral traditions for handling medical-research hazards: the medical-research community itself and the organizations that sponsor human experiments.

I have already identified the scientific community as the carrier of informal morality. Although leaders of the community at large formulate moral traditions, it is often specialized groups within it that negotiate the boundaries between acceptable and unacceptable experiments. Sociologists identify the "problem group" as the basic unit in the organization of scientific work. Problem groups are networks of researchers who address common questions, share materials and techniques, review one another's scientific papers, and debate the meaning of empirical findings.[28] These groups also make consequential judgments about the nature and magnitude of experimental benefits and hazards. Members have the technical knowledge to make moral discriminations on the basis of their own experience with the methods and materials used in generating scientific evidence.

The organizational sponsors of human experiments are another locus of deliberations concerning the acceptability of research hazards. In the United States, clinical investigators have received support for their work from a variety of organizations. These include private research institutes, federal agencies, philanthropic societies, public health departments, and pharmaceutical companies. Some sponsors are the scientist's employer; others are a source of outside funding. In either case, sponsors' control over resources gives them leverage to sustain moral judgments that problem groups, because of their informal nature, typically lack. Both research networks and sponsors weigh the benefits and risks of human experiments. In doing so, they are responsive not only to scientific assessments but also to a range of factors in the broader organizational and cultural environment. In short, moral decisions are social in character both because groups and organizations frame and debate the moral issues and because a variety of social factors shape the outcome of their deliberations.

Collective decision making about investigatory risks is seldom readily apparent from the formal record of science. Professional journals provide abundant evidence of scientific disputes but reveal little about organizational or group dynamics affecting the construction of experimental benefits and hazards. To explore these social processes, I draw upon unpublished archival documents, particularly correspondence between medical researchers and records of organizations supporting clinical experiments. Combined with scientific publications and secondary historical accounts, these documents reveal how research communities and sponsors evaluated and managed investigatory hazards and what factors shaped their judgments about the acceptability of human experiments. Available sources on the use of new vaccines in humans include a rich array of both published and unpublished materials.

Why Vaccine Research?

Several features of vaccine research—apart from the richness of available sources—make it a promising locale for studying clinical investigators' moral traditions. For one, the introduction of new immunizing agents has been accompanied by especially stark discussions of hazards and benefits.

The history of vaccine use is accompanied by an equally long history of vaccine-related deaths and serious injuries. These accidents—as researchers call them—are related to both the contents of immunizing products and the techniques used in creating them. Vaccines are composed of deliberately altered disease-causing microorganisms. Medical researchers produce vaccines by weakening bacteria or viruses so that the altered disease agents will stimulate immunity in human recipients without producing clinical symptoms of illness. Through the mid-twentieth century, scientists used three principal methods for modifying disease agents: physical treatment, chemical treatment, and serial passage through experimental animals—although the last method, in some cases, increases rather than decreases virulence. The resulting immunizing agents were either attenuated or killed.

Vaccine accidents have a number of causes. Some mishaps have occurred when an insufficiently weakened immunizing agent generated cases of the disease that the vaccine was designed to prevent. In some cases, toxic chemical contaminants have sickened vaccine recipients. In others, biological contaminants have caused diseases unrelated to the vaccine's intended composition. In still others, vaccine preparations have triggered acute allergic reactions. These have ranged from temporary inflammation to permanent neurological impairments—including paralysis—and anaphylactic shock, a condition involving systemic failure and rapid death.

While knowledge of vaccine hazards is widespread today, this was not always the case. Graham Wilson, British bacteriologist and author of the 1967 volume *Hazards of Immunization,* comments that the majority of vaccine accidents that occurred during the early and middle decades of the twentieth century went unreported in both the news media and professional journals. Wilson gained access to unpublished public health data while gathering material for his book and was surprised to learn of the large number of people who had died from attempted vaccinations.[29] But if researchers were unaware of the extent of vaccine-related mortality, they were fully cognizant of the varieties of vaccine hazards and their potential seriousness.

Three other features of vaccine research have also encouraged explicit discussion of risks and benefits. First, the recipients of most vaccines are healthy at the time of immunization.[30] Public and professional tolerance for hazards is lower than would be the case if subjects were ill. Second, vaccine recipients are very often children. Youngsters are less likely than adults to have acquired natural immunity to infectious diseases. For this reason, they are both more in need of vaccination and more useful as subjects in immunization research—particularly for studies of vaccine efficacy. The prospect of serious injury to healthy children has meant that the stakes in vaccine debates are particularly high. Third, while the consequences of vaccine accidents can be grave for those harmed, there is clear public interest in employing immunizing agents for control of epidemic disease. In discussions of vaccine use, tension over the priority of individuals' well-being and common social good has been especially strong. Furthermore, vaccine debates have not been restricted to professional communities. In part because the state has an interest in vaccine use, controversies have spilled over into public arenas.

Another reason that vaccine research is an auspicious arena for studying moral traditions is that it has an especially long historical trajectory.[31] Vaccines were among the first clinical innovations developed by laboratory researchers when experimental medicine emerged as a distinct arena of scientific activity during the late nineteenth century. Louis Pasteur introduced several animal vaccines in the late 1870s and early 1880s. With the administration of his rabies vaccine in 1885, he was also the first to inaugurate use of a laboratory-generated immunizing agent in humans. The pace of vaccine development proceeded rapidly in the years that followed. By 1900, scientists had initiated human vaccines against typhoid, cholera, and plague. Before 1930, immunizing agents available for human use included preparations against tuberculosis, diphtheria, tetanus, and pertussis. Some of the early vaccines stimulated immunity, not to the disease-causing microorganism, but to bacterial toxins secondary to infection. The diphtheria and tetanus vaccines were toxoid preparations.

In addition to vaccines, early-twentieth-century researchers introduced a variety of immune sera designed to bolster recipients' immunity through the infusion of antibodies from the blood of convalescing animals or human patients. Scientists referred to the protection that sera afforded as passive immunity, in contrast to the active immunity generated by vaccines, which trigger the body's own production of antibodies. Passive immunity is limited in duration. But before the availability of antibiotics, physicians used serum preparations widely for the treatment and prevention of life-threatening infectious diseases. One of the first serum preparations was diphtheria antitoxin, distributed beginning in the 1890s before the development of diphtheria toxoid. Early-twentieth-century serum products also included preparations against paralytic poliomyelitis.

Researchers have experimented with human applications of laboratory-generated vaccines and sera for well over a century. But human testing of immunizing agents extends back even further than the late nineteenth century. Medical innovators introduced procedures for vaccinating against one epidemic disease, smallpox, long before the advent of modern laboratory sciences. Edward Jenner announced his method for vaccination against smallpox in 1798. Conventional wisdom provided inspiration for Jenner's method. Farmers had long observed that individuals who developed lesions of cowpox after exposure to infected livestock never subsequently contracted smallpox, a much more virulent illness. Jenner's procedure involved deliberately exposing individuals to material extracted from cowpox pustules. Contemporary medical societies endorsed vaccination, and it was widely adopted as a public health measure during the first half of the nineteenth century.

Even Jenner's vaccination did not inaugurate the use of immunizing agents in humans. Vaccination had supplanted a still earlier procedure, inoculation, which involved exposing individuals to material taken from human smallpox pustules. When successful, inoculation resulted in a mild case of smallpox and resistance to subsequent infection. Advocates argued that the procedure was warranted because death rates associated with inoculated smallpox were substantially lower than mortality from naturally contracted smallpox. Introduced to Europe and America in the 1720s, inoculation generated recurring controversy during much of the eighteenth century. Thus, the use of immunizing agents and debates about the acceptability of its human hazards have been ongoing for nearly three centuries. The expanse of this history means that immunization provides an unusual opportunity for exploring the origins of researchers' indigenous morality.

In the course of this volume, I explore the moral discourse surrounding the introduction of smallpox inoculation in the eighteenth century, smallpox vaccine in the nineteenth century, rabies vaccine in the 1880s, influenza vaccines in the 1930s, measles vaccines in the 1940s, and polio vaccines the 1930s and 1950s. The resulting narrative is not a history of immunology or vaccine research. Immunizing agents omitted from the account are many times more numerous than those included. Instead, deliberations over vaccine use are occasions for examining the nature and sources of traditions for handling medical-research hazards and the social processes shaping their implementation. Moreover, in the final chapters of the book, I expand the empirical focus and discuss a broader range of human experiments.

The moral debates examined in this book span more than two centuries, and the professional communities involved in these controversies were by no means equivalent. Two points of divergence include the institutional context of investigatory work and the research community's relation to the practicing branch of medicine. The clarity of demarcations between the two groups has varied in different locations and historical periods. For the purpose of this book, I use the terms "medical scientist," " medical researcher," "medical investigator," and "clinical researcher" interchangeably to refer to someone who undertook human experiments or who evaluated empirical data on the safety and efficacy of a clinical innovation. I use the term "physician," when not further qualified, to refer to someone whose primary affiliation was with the practicing branch of the profession.

Perspectives and Themes

The approach of this book cuts across disciplines. I address issues with immediate and practical implications for bioethics and science policy. I use the primary data of a historian while drawing concepts and perspectives from the field of sociology. Moral decision making in medicine has become a burgeoning arena of sociological study. In recent years, scholars have employed ethnographic and other qualitative techniques to examine social factors that shape the framing and outcome of moral decisions in clinical settings. Their work reveals that organizational and occupational processes powerfully influence how health care providers define moral issues and act on these constructions.[32] My analysis expands the purview of this dynamic arena of study both by considering historical patterns in moral decision making and by addressing dilemmas in the introduction of risk-laden medical technologies. In doing so, I borrow from—and draw links between—multiple perspectives in the discipline of sociology.

In chapters 1 and 2, I examine the research community as the bearer of moral oversight. Chapter 1 follows a sequence of historical episodes in which the professionals inaugurating and evaluating new immunizing agents gave expression to a moral logic of risk. These episodes—extending from the third decade of the eighteenth century to the early 1900s—shed light on the origins and character of traditions for conducting human trials and the purposes these traditions have served. Chapter 2 recounts a single episode in 1934–35 in which American scientists stopped the use of two polio vaccines that the research community decided were overly hazardous. Here I underscore both the complexities that arise when investigators apply their traditions to specific cases and the strengths and weaknesses of the research network as a locus for moral oversight. My analysis in these chapters incorporates major concepts from the sociology of science: the problem group as the basic unit in the organization of research communities; the "gift culture" of science that generates collegial exchanges; and "local knowledge"—hands-on experience with materials and methods—that is key to researchers' evaluations of empirical findings. These notions clarify the scientific debates to which researchers' moral assessments are integrally tied.

My focus in chapters 3 and 4 is the oversight exercised by the organizations that sponsored clinical research. Chapter 3 explores differences in sponsors' approaches to hazards. By comparing vaccine trials, I show that some organizations were risk adverse and others tolerant when confronting very similar hazards. Chapter 4 addresses trends over time in sponsors' policies toward risk. Extending my empirical scope beyond vaccine testing, I present evidence that, between the mid-1930s and mid-1950s, several major sponsors were adopting a common set of procedures for managing hazards and, in doing so, constructing a rudimentary oversight system. In these chapters, I bring to bear two major ideas from the sociology of organizations: that interactions with the environment importantly affect organizational policies and that organizations tend to import legitimacy-conferring models from professions and the law. These notions help to explain both difference between and growing similarities in sponsors' stances toward risk.

In chapter 5, I discuss long-term patterns in the oversight of human research and the relation of early moral traditions and organizational procedures to the government regulation inaugurated in the 1960s. I also discuss the contributions of my historical analysis to sociological theory. Chapter 6 serves as an epilogue, clarifying implications of the book's findings for understanding recent regulatory failures. My focus here concerns events surrounding the death of two research subjects in experiments conducted during the late 1990s and early 2000s. I argue that moral traditions are not merely relics of the past. They continue to operate today and have immediate relevance for the design of federally mandated research oversight.

Three themes unify the various threads of my analysis. The first bears on the capacity of scientific communities to constrain the conduct of their members. While medical researchers have well-established moral traditions, the colleague network alone has serious limitations as a site for regulating investigatory hazards. Social processes affect how scientists apply their moral logic and the results have often fallen short of protecting human subjects.

A second theme concerns the importance of outside audiences to researchers' calculations about the assumption of risk. The need to maintain social legitimacy has powerfully influenced how both scientific communities and their sponsors manage hazards and where they draw boundaries between acceptable and unacceptable experiments. Research risks are a problem at two levels. They are threats to the well-being of human subjects who might incur injury. Hazards are also threats to institutions of science because, if human injury does occur, investigatory communities and their

sponsors may encounter challenges to their authority, the withdrawal of resources, and calls for the external regulation of research. Both scientists and
sponsors thus must manage the pursuit of benefits and hazards so as to sustain their legitimacy with outside audiences.[33] Medical innovators have had
two major responses to problems of legitimacy. They have been highly alert
to public attitudes, with the result that the prevailing cultural climate has
importantly affected the level and type of hazards investigators have assumed. Meanwhile, both research communities and their sponsors have devoted substantial resources to shaping popular constructions of risk.

A final theme relates to the emergence of systems for overseeing technological hazards. I argue that, over time, research oversight has became
more formal and more institutionally embedded, and that a variety of social
processes have fostered long-term change. My analysis of these processes
sheds light not only on the regulation of human research but also on the
management, more broadly, of socially desirable but potentially dangerous
products of modern science.

1

The Origins of a Moral Logic of Risk

Medical-research communities have longstanding traditions for handling the risks that human experiments entail. A cornerstone of these traditions is the logic of lesser harms, whereby hazardous interventions are moral if they generate net benefit and the risks are lower than those of the natural disease. Four other expectations have accompanied lesser-harm reasoning: researchers require that animal tests precede human experiments; they delay or suspend human use if the hazards of a procedure appear too grave; they insist that only scientifically sound experiments are moral, because bad research cannot contribute to the common good; and many have begun human testing by first experimenting on themselves. Evidence for these traditions can be found in the work of historians and ethnographers who study medical researchers and in the statements and actions of clinical investigators, present and past.

Modern communities of medical researchers—investigators devoted to developing and testing new medical interventions—did not coalesce until the second half of the nineteenth century. Before then, a variety of professional groups were instrumental in inaugurating new medical procedures, including natural scientists and empirically minded physicians. These early medical innovators also observed a moral logic of risk.

In this chapter, I examine historical episodes in which those initiating and studying medical innovations articulated or displayed their moral logic with clarity. Members of social groups often find it difficult to put words to their informal norms and customs. The professionals introducing new

medical procedures were no exception in this regard. Their rules for conducting human experiments often remained tacit or only partly articulated.
But periodically, medical innovators made cohesive statements of their
moral reasoning. Members of a fledgling scientific community articulated
lesser-harm logic in early-eighteenth-century debates over smallpox inoculation. Empirically minded physicians and public health advocates invoked
lesser-harm reasoning in nineteenth-century disputes over smallpox vaccination. Supporters and leaders of the new laboratory medicine asserted the
importance of animal experimentation—and by extension, clinical moratoria—in the 1880s, during controversy surrounding the use of Pasteur's rabies vaccine. Early in the twentieth century, spokesmen for the emerging
medical-research community in America gave voice to a full range of moral
traditions when responding to the allegations of antivivisection activists.

My analysis of these episodes sheds light on the character of experimenters' informal morality and the purposes their moral logic has served. I
argue that traditions for conducting human experiments are, in large measure, an outgrowth of the cognitive norms of science. But when medical innovators give voice to their traditions, it has often been to serve social ends.
Experimenters' moral traditions have been a set of standards for decisions
about proceeding with human experiments. They have also provided rhetorical tools for justifying both clinical use of hazardous medical interventions
and the pursuit of medical science itself.

Before I proceed, several caveats are in order. I am not attempting here to
provide a comprehensive history of traditions for handling experimental
or otherwise risky medical interventions. There are undoubtedly many occasions, unexamined in the pages below, in which scientists give voice to
their moral traditions. Nor is it my intention, in noting similarities across
episodes, to obscure important differences in the groups undertaking vaccine innovation. The communities that inaugurated use of different immunizing agents were by no means the same. Furthermore, while physicians
were among the early medical innovators, those introducing new procedures were often at odds with the practicing branch of the medical profession. There were fundamental tensions between the research and practicing
segments of medicine and, to a considerable degree, these persist today.[1]

Finally, in pointing to historical antecedents of twentieth-century investigatory morality, I am not suggesting that expressions of normative traditions have the same meaning for early innovators and later generations of
researchers. Periodic changes occur in the institutions of science and in the
dominant paradigms and methods that help shape its content. Moral traditions are bound to have different meanings for investigators who work in

disparate professional contexts. Such differences notwithstanding, a clear pattern emerges from the historical record: later medical researchers borrowed freely from the conceptual and linguistic formulations of experimenters who preceded them. The discourse of early medical innovators was a cultural resource for subsequent generations of scientists.

The Logic of Lesser Harms

Eighteenth- and nineteenth-century professional communities articulated lesser-harm logic in a series of controversies over the use of immunizing agents. During the 1720s, members and supporters of the earliest scientific associations—societies founded in Europe during the second half of the seventeenth century—invoked lesser-harm logic when promoting smallpox inoculation. They sought to address public fears about the hazards of inoculation and to demonstrate the social utility of the new empirical science. In the nineteenth century, public health advocates borrowed from the same moral tradition when constructing arguments supporting compulsory vaccination.

Marshaling Evidence for Smallpox Inoculation

In the early decades of the eighteenth century, the newly established scientific societies of Europe took up the matter of smallpox inoculation. In Britain, physicians and surgeons who supported the scientific movement introduced inoculation in the early 1720s. Members of the Royal Society of London (constituted in the early 1660s) oversaw early inoculations and undertook the collection of evidence on the procedure's effectiveness and safety. Proponents of the new science among the educated classes encouraged these activities. In France, opposition from the conservative medical establishment delayed the use of inoculation until the 1750s. There midcentury advocates for the procedure included royalty, court physicians, scientists in the Académie Royale des Sciences, and many among *les philosophes*—intellectuals who championed Enlightenment thought.[2]

The association of smallpox inoculation with modern science is not without irony. Inoculation was by no means a product of Western scientific discovery. The procedure had arrived in Europe and America from the East—China, India, Persia, Turkey—where it had long flourished as a medical practice. But to champions of the natural philosophy sweeping contemporary European thought, inoculation exemplified the social benefits of empirical inquiry. Scientists and their supporters declared that judgments about the procedure should be based upon systematic observation. They defended their position in debates that became highly visible through a series of pamphlet wars.

Inoculation generated opposition on both religious and medical grounds. Conservative theologians argued that the procedure usurped Providence, promoting vice and immorality. Medical practitioners raised several objections. Some questioned whether it was moral to deliberately inflict a disease even if the result was protection from a more serious affliction. (Successful inoculation resulted in a mild case of smallpox. While most inoculated cases were less serious than natural smallpox, deaths from smallpox did occur among the inoculated.) Other physicians doubted that inoculated smallpox would consistently protect against the natural disease. Still others speculated that the procedure might induce serious diseases other than smallpox—contemporary medical theory held that the state of the blood at the time of infection determined what type of illness a person contracted. Pamphlets distributed by the opposition fanned widespread fears about the dangers of the new procedure.[3]

Proponents of inoculation avoided debating religion or medical theory. They insisted that decisions about the procedure's use be grounded not on public fears, religious doctrine, or medical theory, but rather upon observation and reason. For the scientific community, inoculation was an occasion for applying empirical methods of natural philosophy to a matter of social importance and for demonstrating that these methods had practical utility.

British empiricists pursued two approaches when applying methods of the new science. First, they conducted experimental demonstrations of inoculation, witnessed by the broader community of scientists. Then they collected and reported numerical evidence on the relative probabilities of death from natural and inoculated smallpox. The second approach would involve the calculation of lesser harms.

The most highly visible experiment took place at London's Newgate Prison in August 1721. With the permission of the king, surgeon Charles Maitland inoculated six prisoners who had been condemned to die. Two court physicians oversaw Maitland's prison inoculations. One was Sir Hans Sloane, a fellow of the Royal Society and a leading promoter of the new science. Twenty-five witnesses attended the demonstration, including prominent members of the Royal Society and Royal College of Physicians. Announcements issued prior to the experiment invited interested parties not only to attend the procedures but also to visit the prisoners in the weeks following their inoculations. The results of the experiment were auspicious. Of the six inmates, five contracted mild cases of smallpox and quickly recovered. One, previously afflicted with natural smallpox, had no reaction to the procedure.[4]

Shortly after the Newgate demonstration, scientists began collecting data on the relative harms of inoculated and natural smallpox. James Jurin was the chief chronicler of numerical evidence. Jurin was a physician, mathematician, and secretary to the Royal Society between 1722 and 1727, under Isaac Newton's presidency. During his tenure as secretary, Jurin compiled yearly reports on the mortality rates of natural and inoculated smallpox. These accounts addressed two questions: Did inoculation provide genuine security against natural smallpox? And were the hazards of the procedure lower than the risks of the naturally contracted disease? Jurin's results appeared in the Royal Society's publication *Philosophical Transactions* and as separately bound, and widely distributed, offprints.[5]

Historian Andrea Rusnock details the methods Jurin used to compile evidence. For information on inoculated smallpox, he drew on a wide-ranging network of correspondents. By letter, Jurin solicited and received data on the numbers and results of inoculation. He took great care in assessing the reliability of his informants' testimony. He investigated ambiguous cases and refuted what he judged to be false accounts of negative outcomes. Jurin based his early calculations of mortality from natural smallpox on the London bills of mortality, which had been instituted in the 1660s to track outbreaks of epidemic diseases. He also received reports from his correspondents on natural-smallpox mortality within communities experiencing epidemics.[6] Jurin thus functioned as an informal clearinghouse for national and international communications on the status of inoculation, not only soliciting information, but also making his accumulated knowledge available in response to outside inquiries. He exchanged information with scientific societies on the Continent and received reports on inoculation from as far away as Boston.[7]

The outcome of Jurin's inquiries was favorable for the subsequent adoption of inoculation. He found no instances where successful inoculation—indicated by a distinctive lesion at the point of incision and a mild case of smallpox—failed to provide protection against the natural disease. Regarding relative hazards, Jurin reported that inoculated smallpox carried a substantially lower risk of mortality than naturally contracted smallpox. In 1728, a colleague of Jurin's updated the Royal Society's reports of inoculations performed in the British Isles, Germany, and America. The accumulated record included 845 cases of inoculated smallpox with 17 fatalities. This yielded a death rate of 1 in 50 cases. In contrast, the death rate for natural smallpox was approximately 1 in 6 cases.[8] The implication was clear: inoculation yielded undoubted benefit and its risks were discernibly lower than the hazards of the natural disease.

The inoculation controversy in early-eighteenth-century Britain sheds light on both the conditions giving rise to lesser-harm reasoning and the purposes to which the logic was put. Several historical developments made the calculation of lesser harms possible. For one thing, growing use of inoculation allowed its clinical outcomes to be studied. Following the Newgate demonstrations and several other experiments, upper-class parents in Britain began to inoculate their children in small but growing numbers.[9] Lesser-harm formulations, when based on human-use data, are inevitably post hoc arguments.[10] Another factor making calculations like Jurin's feasible was the availability of numerical evidence on fatalities from natural smallpox. As already mentioned, in the London bills of mortality, scientists had access to data that allowed them to estimate the risk of death from the naturally occurring disease. Still another factor was the development of the field of mathematics then called probability. While Jurin used simple arithmetic in calculating the relative risks of dying from natural and inoculated smallpox, the availability of probability theory undoubtedly fostered his adoption of a mathematical approach to the problem.[11]

Most important for the present argument, Jurin and his colleagues drew upon prevailing notions about the conduct of scientific inquiry. Both experimental demonstrations and the calculation of lesser harms had roots in contemporary beliefs about how to ascertain matters of fact. Seventeenth-century empiricists adopted the view that, because knowledge of the physical world can be derived only through experience, truths concerning natural sciences are unavoidably provisional and revisable. From this perspective, arriving at shared understandings about experimental truths was inherently problematic. Steven Shapin and Simon Schaffer argue that scientists developed a number of strategies for authenticating knowledge and generating agreements about what constitutes a scientific fact. These strategies included conducting experiments in public space (including the laboratory), securing multiple witnesses to publicly announced experimental demonstrations, and invoking the testimony of observers deemed reliable and trustworthy. Collective witnessing served to correct for individual bias and differences in observational ability.[12]

Like experimental demonstrations, mathematical calculation of lesser harms was compatible with prevailing strategies for discerning empirical truths. Contemporary natural philosophy viewed knowledge in the sciences as inherently probabilistic. Basing determinations of fact upon observation and experience left findings vulnerable to human fallibility. The best one could hope for when apprehending the natural world was a high degree of probability. British scientists applied mathematical—and probabilistic—analysis to a wide range of phenomena.[13]

If the calculation of relative harms was a means for determining matters of fact, it was also a vehicle for programmatic argument. Jurin and his colleagues invoked lesser-harm reasoning in response to critics and detractors of inoculation. The Royal Society's numerical evidence on benefits and hazards of inoculation was crucial to the growing acceptance of the procedure in eighteenth-century Europe.[14] Contemporary tributes to Jurin's work acknowledged the practical ends of lesser-harm calculations. John Woodhouse, a physician from Nottingham, wrote to Jurin in 1726:

> Hearty thanks for your good Intentions to the Publick by continuing This Annuall Account which will I doubt not soon Convince all Enemys to this Practice and Establish it for the Great Benefit of Mankind.[15]

Recent work by historians suggests that, during the late seventeenth and early eighteenth centuries, science became an increasingly vital part of public culture.[16] The educated public took unprecedented interest in empirical findings, and science had a growing impact on public consciousness and governmental policies. For the emerging research community, lesser-harm calculations were a means for asserting the legitimacy of science as a public asset. Their formulations provided evidence for both the merits of inoculation and the social utility of empirical science.

Individual or Collective Good?

Jurin's calculations did not end controversy over the risks and benefits of smallpox inoculation. Between 1750 and 1770, heated debate took place in Europe over the advisability of adopting the procedure. Meanwhile, a disagreement arose within intellectual circles over the use of lesser-harm reasoning. In 1760, the Swiss mathematician Daniel Bernoulli and French philosopher Jean D'Alembert debated the terms of the lesser-harm calculus in treatises delivered to the Académie Royale des Sciences in Paris.[17] The controversy originated in observations made by Charles Marie de La Condamine, a leading figure in the Académie Royale, about limitations to the lesser-harm formulations published by the Royal Society in Britain. La Condamine was a proponent of inoculation and—much as Jurin had been a generation earlier—a center for scientific communication about the procedure. La Condamine argued that Jurin, in comparing mortality from natural and inoculated smallpox, had failed to take into account that not all individuals would contract natural smallpox. At issue, in La Condamine's view, was not the relative mortality rates but, rather, how individuals should weigh the short-term risk of dying from inoculated smallpox against the long-term risk of both contracting and succumbing to natural smallpox.

Bernoulli pursued La Condamine's formulation in a memoir read to the Académie Royale in April 1760 and published in 1766. This paper was a mathematical treatise on the relative hazards of inoculated and natural smallpox. Bernoulli provided no new data. He based his computations on existing estimates of smallpox morbidity and mortality. What he offered was a new application of probability theory, one that took into account the risks of contracting natural smallpox. Bernoulli's approach was to calculate average life expectancies of both individuals who had and those who had not been inoculated. His calculations showed average gains in life expectancy when inoculation was performed at various ages. Bernoulli concluded that inoculation offered substantial net benefit: individuals who chose inoculation lived, on average, three years longer than those who took their chances with natural smallpox.

D'Alembert responded with his own treatise, delivered in November of 1760. His presentation faulted Bernoulli's calculations on two grounds. First, available evidence on morbidity and mortality from natural and inoculated smallpox was meager, an insufficient basis for decisions about the wisdom of inoculation. Second, Bernoulli had left out of his calculations the individual's perceptions of the relative importance of short-term risk and long-term hazards. D'Alembert insisted on the primacy of the individual's perceptions and experiences. Most people, he argued, would rather take their chances with a danger that might strike at some time in the future than willingly subject themselves to an immediate hazard, albeit one that is smaller.

The dispute between Bernoulli and D'Alembert had implications for the use of lesser-harm formulations in programmatic argument. La Condamine and his followers insisted that inoculation was in the public good and that the state had an interest in promoting its use. They made this argument on both humanitarian and economic grounds. State support for inoculation would save lives and, and by doing so, enhance the nation's wealth.[18] D'Alembert's position suggested that it was inappropriate to use lesser-harm formulations in a programmatic argument. In this view, decisions about the use of inoculation should be based not on notions about the common good or the interests of the state—or on scientists' calculations of a person's probable best interests—but rather on the individual's perceptions of and preferences about risks.[19]

In the decades that followed, lesser-harm reasoning remained central to professional debates over immunization policies. Over time, it would also become a prominent feature of debates taking place within public arenas. The disagreement between Bernoulli and D'Alembert was one in a long series of controversies concerning the terms of the lesser-harm calculus and its use in public health controversies. Many of these later disputes would also involve competing notions about the relative value of individual prerogatives and the common good, and about the definition and measurement of benefits and harms.

The Politics of Smallpox Vaccination

During the first half of the nineteenth century, vaccination replaced inoculation as the preferred method for immunizing against smallpox. The new procedure exposed recipients to cowpox or its derivatives, immunologically similar to smallpox but considerably less virulent. Following the 1798 publication of Edward Jenner's inquiry, which presented case histories of twenty-three patients vaccinated with smallpox, a flurry of additional studies of the procedure appeared in the medical literature.[20] It was quickly apparent that vaccination produced immunity while generating milder symptoms, fewer complications, and substantially lower mortality than inoculated smallpox. Furthermore, in contrast to inoculation, individuals immunized with cowpox were not contagious to those around them. Proponents of vaccination used lesser-harm reasoning when evaluating the new method for protecting against smallpox. But they now adjusted the reasoning to accommodate the existence of the established immunization procedure. In this modified form, lesser-harm logic placed as much emphasis on comparing the dangers of vaccination to those of the older intervention as to those of the disease itself.[21]

Initial debates about vaccination were confined largely to the scientific and medical communities. Medical practitioners had a variety of concerns about the new method. Some objected to both inoculation and vaccination, pointing to the secondary infections that immunization could generate.[22] Others continued to prefer inoculation, questioning the ability of vaccination to confer life-long protection. A number of physicians argued that early vaccinators had contaminated their cowpox samples with natural smallpox and were, in reality, immunizing with attenuated smallpox.[23] Whatever the actual composition of the new immunizing agent, the adoption of vaccination proceeded rapidly and with the support of the medical establishment. The Royal College of Physicians formally endorsed the procedure in 1807.

That year, London's Inoculation Hospital abandoned inoculation in favor of vaccination for outpatients; in 1821, the hospital stopped performing inoculation in-house. British law made inoculation illegal in 1840, and during the following year, Parliament made free vaccinations available through the Poor Law authorities.

After midcentury, the character of the vaccination controversy changed dramatically. Britain's Vaccination Act of 1853 made childhood immunization against smallpox mandatory. What had been a debate within professional communities now spilled into public arenas. Initially the law was not enforced. But legislation enacted in the late 1860s and early 1870s created a mechanism for punishing violators. In 1871, spurred in part by an outbreak of smallpox, Parliament mandated that the government's recently authorized vaccination officers could fine and, ultimately, imprison noncompliant parents. Compulsory vaccination triggered heated public controversy. An anti-vaccination movement coalesced in the 1870s and burgeoned during the final decades of the century. It led to sporadic protests, debates in the press, the proliferation of anti-vaccination societies, and increasingly well organized efforts to influence public opinion and government policy.

I cannot do justice here to the complexities of the late-nineteenth-century vaccination debates and their relation to medical theory and national politics in Britain.[24] I focus in this discussion on features of the controversy with particular relevance to the social uses of lesser-harm reasoning. On this matter, three points are noteworthy. First, both supporters and detractors of vaccination invoked lesser-harm logic and marshaled numerical evidence in support of their arguments. The Epidemiological Society, an advocate of mandatory vaccination, produced regular reports on deaths from smallpox. Its figures revealed substantially lower rates of smallpox mortality among those undergoing vaccination. Opponents compiled their own numbers, and these showed no net benefit from vaccination. The editor of a leading movement publication, *Vaccination Inquirer,* insisted that there was no statistical proof that vaccination provided protection against either contracting or dying from smallpox. The *Inquirer* and other anti-vaccination outlets engaged in "statistical warfare against pro-vaccinationism."[25] A long-term decline in the incidence of smallpox complicated the debate. Vaccination proponents attributed this trend to the widespread adoption of the procedure; detractors attributed it to improved sanitation and other public health measures.

Second, tension between the common good and individual liberty was at the core of public controversy over vaccination policy. Supporters of mandatory vaccination argued that the measure would lessen both human misery and damage to the nation's physical and economic health. Those holding liberal political views maintained that it was appropriate for government to regulate individual liberties in ways consistent with social progress.[26] In contrast, opponents considered mandatory vaccination an intolerable obstacle to freedom of conscience. In the end, Parliament abandoned compulsory vaccination. Historian Anne Hardy writes that "it was England's deep-rooted individualism that ultimately brought the state's withdrawal" from mandatory immunization.[27] It undoubtedly helped also that, after the smallpox outbreak in 1871 and subsequent vaccination measures, new cases of the disease became less and less common. In the late 1890s, Parliament scaled down its vaccination-enforcement measures and instituted provisions for conscientious objectors to childhood immunization. In 1907, it withdrew from setting immunization policy altogether, delegating this and other public health matters to local health departments and professional societies.

Finally, in these vaccination debates, the logic and language of risks and benefits emerged as a routine and expected feature of public-policy discourse. In 1889, Parliament appointed the Royal Commission on Vaccination to assess criticisms of state policy and make recommendations about the future of vaccination laws. The commission's final report, published in 1898, made numerous concessions to opponents of vaccination. But the majority report was a pro-vaccination statement, and its text provides numerous examples of lesser-harm reasoning as a tool for persuasion. The authors acknowledged that in a small number of cases, "injury and death [had] resulted from vaccination." But they insisted that the procedure's "substantial benefit in limiting the ravages of smallpox" greatly outweighed its harms.[28] The hazards of vaccination were not only small in relation to the benefits, they were also, in themselves, negligible. The authors included a narrative on the hazards of modern life that served to normalize vaccine risks by comparing them to dangers of other commonly used and socially desirable technologies:

> Danger of personal injury, and even of death, attends many of the most common incidents of life, but experience has shown the risk to be so small that it is every day disregarded. A railway journey or a walk in the streets of any large town certainly involves such risks, but they are not deemed serious enough to induce anyone to refrain from traveling or from frequenting the public streets. And to come within the region of therapeutics, it cannot be denied that a risk attaches in every case where chloroform is administered [as an anesthetic]; it is nevertheless constantly resorted to, where the

only object is to escape temporary pain. The admission, therefore, that
some risk attaches to the operation of vaccination, an admission which
must without hesitation be made, does not necessarily afford an argument
of any cogency against the practice, if its consequences be on the whole
beneficial and important, the risk may be so small that it is reasonable to
disregard it.[29]

This logic was clearly applicable to other medical procedures and, indeed, to
a broad range of technical innovations. Compulsory vaccination was no
longer an issue in Britain by the early 1900s. But the example of risk-benefit
reasoning promoting public acceptance of a potentially hazardous technology remained as a cultural resource.

Legacies of Laboratory Medicine: Moratoria and Animal Testing

While participants in British immunization debates were marshaling lesser-
harm arguments for and against compulsory vaccination, laboratory researchers on the Continent were generating a different type of moral discourse. At issue was how laboratory-generated medical innovations would
be introduced into clinical practice. Two interrelated practices would be central to handling the risks that such innovations entailed: animal testing and
delaying human use until the safety of an intervention had been demonstrated in the laboratory. Scientists affirmed their commitment to these
measures during the 1880s in discussions of Pasteur's rabies vaccine. At
first, they directed their discourse on these practices toward the scientific
and medical communities.

Laboratory medicine emerged as a distinct arena of research in the final
third of the nineteenth century. During the 1860s and 1870s, scientists in
France and Germany developed methods for observing, isolating, and cultivating microorganisms. Their efforts yielded both systematic evidence for
the germ theory of disease and improved capabilities for identifying the bacteriological agents causing specific infectious illnesses. Contemporary scientists announced the discovery of microorganisms responsible for a growing number of epidemic diseases. Among them was the bacterium causing
tuberculosis, a leading source of mortality in the late nineteenth century,
isolated by Robert Koch in 1882. Meanwhile, Pasteur had been developing
methods for attenuating bacteria and for generating disease immunity
through the application of laboratory-altered microorganisms. In 1881, he
demonstrated the protective effects of a laboratory-generated anthrax vaccine in an experiment with sheep. Extrapolating from these events, propo-

nents of scientific medicine argued that laboratory research was on the verge of yielding tools for creating human immunity to a host of life-threatening infectious diseases.

Less than two weeks after Koch announced that he had isolated the tuberculosis bacterium, the London *Times* ran an editorial on the implications of his discovery. The *Times* statement is remarkable both for its accessible explanation of immunization and its confidence that an effective vaccine against tuberculosis would soon be available.[30] In fact, it would be forty years before researchers succeeded in developing a vaccine for tuberculosis that was sufficiently effective and safe for human use.[31] According to the *Times* of April 22, 1882:

> If Dr. Koch's investigations and conclusions should be confirmed by further experiments, we shall be able to entertain a reasonable hope that an antidote to consumption and to tuberculous diseases generally may at a not distant date be brought within our reach. It is characteristic of many of the disease-producing bacilli, and probably of all of them, that they can be so altered by cultivation as to produce a mild disease instead of a severe one, and that the designed communication of the former will afford protection against the latter. Pasteur has lately shown how completely this may be accomplished in the case of the bacillus which causes [anthrax]; and [smallpox] vaccination itself is now regarded merely as inoculation with the smallpox bacillus, after this had been modified in its character by being cultivated in the bodies of the bovine race. The experiments of Dr. Koch . . . seem as yet to have been carried not further than to the repeated cultivation of the tubercule bacillis in its original virulence; but they will speedily be followed, as a matter of course, by attempts at cultivation in diminished intensity.[32]

At least one newspaper in the United States carried similar commentary. A statement in the *New York Tribune* on May 3, 1882, echoed the *Times* editorial:

> It is a well appreciated fact that parasites which produce analogous diseases in animals and in the human system can be modified by cultivation until they finally produce a mild form of those diseases, and in this way protection may be afforded against virulent conditions. The analogies of diseases imply that it may be possible to procure from guinea-pigs or rabbits an effective inoculant against consumption, precisely as smallpox germs are cultivated in the cow or [anthrax] germs in sheep. It is the possibility of con-

verting the [tuberculosis bacterium] into a prophylactic or preventive agent that lends importance to [Koch's] interesting experiments.[33]

Both researchers and the educated laity anticipated that medical scientists would be developing immunizing agents in the laboratory and introducing these preparations into clinical practice. But how would investigators handle the hazards that such vaccines would entail? Researchers were well aware that risks would accompany human use of laboratory vaccines. Complications and unanticipated diseases had accompanied the adoption of both smallpox inoculation and smallpox vaccination. New vaccines would expose man to disease-causing microbes—albeit in modified forms. How would scientists know whether their preparations were sufficiently weakened and otherwise sufficiently safe to avoid human injury? Pasteur's rabies vaccine was the first laboratory-generated immunizing agent to proceed to human testing. Discourse surrounding its early clinical use reveals scientists' standards for the moral conduct of human experiments with such preparations.

Pasteur's team conducted the first human inoculations with rabies vaccine during the summer and fall of 1885. The initial recipients were nine-year-old Joseph Meister, vaccinated in July, and fifteen-year-old Jean-Baptiste Jupille, in October.[34] Both boys were victims of bites by rabid dogs—rabies is one of the few vaccines administered after rather than before exposure to infection.[35] Pasteur had no medical degree and was prohibited by law from conducting the procedure. It was a physician colleague of Pasteur's, Jacques-Joseph Grancher, who performed the series of injections for each of the patients.

Significantly, in the months preceding the vaccinations, Pasteur had made repeated statements about the need for numerous animal trials before his vaccine could be administered to human recipients. Pasteur's frequent and adamant statements are especially interesting in light of Gerald Geison's discoveries in *The Private Science of Louis Pasteur*. Geison examined Pasteur's laboratory notebooks and concluded that the sequence of preparations administered to Meister and Jupille involved a newly developed method, one that Pasteur had previously tested on a relatively small number of animals.[36] In Geison's account, at most twenty dogs had been inoculated by this method. None of these animals had prior exposure to rabies—necessary to assess the technique's efficacy. And at the time of Meister's treatment, inoculation of the twenty dogs was so recent that none had survived as long as thirty days since its final immunization.[37] Pasteur's actual investigatory conduct presented a sharp contrast to his public statements about the need for repeated rounds of animal tests prior to human application. Yet it is clear from his statements that Pasteur was presenting the case that systematic animal experimentation was necessary before the human use of an experimental vaccine was moral. It is clear, also, that the medical researchers and empirically oriented physicians concurred.

Pasteur began his laboratory research on rabies in 1881. His early work focused on techniques for transmitting the disease from animal to animal, first by cerebral and then by intravenous inoculation of infected brain tissue. He then moved to testing a variety of methods for preparing rabies vaccines. In an address delivered at the Académie Royale des Sciences in February 1884, and elaborated in a paper of May 1884, Pasteur announced he had succeeded in making dogs resistant to rabies. He also began making statements about the requirements to be met before human use of a rabies vaccine. For example, when speaking to the International Medical Congress in Copenhagen in August 1884, Pasteur insisted that animal experiments should establish the safety and efficacy of an immunizing agent prior to human application. Furthermore, "proofs must be multiplied *ad infinitum* on diverse animal species before human therapeutics should dare to try this mode of prophylaxis on man himself."[38]

Whether Pasteur had, in fact, been sufficiently systematic in his animal experimentation was the subject of dispute within the professional community. In 1887, the Académie de Médecine held three meetings addressing Pasteur's methods. Much of the discussion concerned several cases in which individuals treated with Pasteur's vaccine subsequently contracted and died of rabies. The implications of these cases for the vaccine's safety and efficacy were at issue. Geison notes that sentiment at the academy meetings was overwhelmingly favorable toward Pasteur's work.[39] Nonetheless, there was dissatisfaction with the small number of animal experiments Pasteur had conducted before initiating human use of his preparation. His most vocal detractor, Michel Peter, complained that Pasteur had not specified precisely how many animals he had inoculated with the preparation before its use with humans, nor had Pasteur described, with any precision, the outcome of these experiments.[40]

Pasteur was absent from these meetings. His compatriots, Grancher and the physiologist Edme Félix Alfred Vulpian, were among those defending his research. During the proceedings, Vulpian declared that criticism from Peter amounted to an accusation of involuntary homicide.[41] But even among Pasteur's supporters, many felt that his method for immunizing against rabies had been inadequately tested. Grancher later recounted a conversation with his colleague Stéphane Tarnier that reveals this undercurrent

of professional dissent. René Dubos, in his biography of Pasteur, quotes
Grancher:

> I can still hear Tarnier speaking, as we walked out of those memorable
> meetings at the Academy of Medicine where Pasteur's adversaries accused
> him and his disciples of homicide. "My dear friend," Tarnier told me, "it
> would be necessary to demonstrate, by repeated experiments, that you can
> cure a dog, even after intracranial inoculation [with rabies-infected cerebral
> material]; that done, you would be left in peace." I replied that these experi-
> ments had been made; but Tarnier did not find them numerous enough,
> and still he was one of Pasteur's friends.[42]

The issue of whether Pasteur had conducted a sufficient number of animal experiments to justify human application was never resolved. Disagreements of this type would recur. Questions concerning the safety of Pasteur's
rabies vaccine also remained.[43] But the importance researchers placed on
animal testing is clear from the debate surrounding the vaccine. A widespread agreement existed among medical researchers and empirically oriented physicians that animal experimentation was a moral imperative before the human testing of a laboratory innovation. Investigators should
refrain from human use of an experimental procedure—that is, they should
observe a clinical moratorium—until problems that might present significant risks to human safety were solved in the laboratory. During the 1880s,
controversy surrounding Pasteur's research remained internal to professional communities.[44] But it would not be long before medical researchers
working in a different setting would invoke the same investigatory practices
in rhetoric directed toward a wider audience.

In Defense of Medical Research

Although European scientists offered some of the earliest expressions of a
moral logic of risk, American medical investigators at the turn of the century
fully embraced the traditions of the broader professional community.
Spokesmen for medical science in the United States made this clear in their
responses to the antivivisection movement of the early 1900s. Antivivisectionists are best known for their opposition to animal research. But the
movement also raised objections to human experimentation, and the moderate antivivisectionist position—that experimentation should be controlled
but not prohibited—generated considerable support from the educated
classes. Scientific leaders sought to neutralize the impact of antivivisection

publicity in part by directing statements of the research community's informal morality toward the public and the rank and file of the medical profession. In doing so, they repeatedly drew from the earlier formulations of their European colleagues.

American science became a presence in the world of biomedical research in the initial decades of the twentieth century.[45] New career tracks in medical research helped foster its growing eminence. With the transformation in American professional colleges during the late nineteenth century, leading medical schools expected faculty to engage in research. Salaried positions for teacher-investigators became increasingly widespread, first in the basic sciences and then within clinical departments.[46] Laboratories at public health agencies and newly established research institutes also provided full-time employment for medical investigators. At the turn of the century, an expanding cadre of American scientists was engaged in basic and applied medical research.

But even as medical science was becoming established within American institutions, the broader medical profession and the public were demonstrating ambivalence about experiments with animals and humans. Antivivisection societies appeared in the United States during the final decades of the nineteenth century, and by the early 1900s, activism against human experimentation gained momentum.[47] Movement leaders generated narratives of investigatory abuses and won coverage for these accounts in the popular press. Their stories discredited nontherapeutic medical research with dramatic portrayals of practices that were cruel or insensitive to subjects. Activists routinely questioned whether participation in even therapeutic research was voluntary—particularly where it involved prisoners, children, or hospitalized patients.

Meanwhile, antivivisection proponents mounted efforts to secure government control of animal and human experimentation. In 1896 and 1900, the U.S. Congress considered a bill that would have regulated animal research within the District of Columbia. During the latter year, Congress also debated legislation aimed at controlling human experimentation in the District. In 1913, following sensational newspaper accounts of research on hospital patients and institutionalized children, advocates persuaded legislators in Pennsylvania to introduce legislation to curtail human experiments not directly related to the subjects' own medical treatment. The following year, U.S. senators sought support for a formal commission to investigate nontherapeutic experiments conducted in public hospitals. The states of New York and New Jersey considered similar bills. The antivivisectionists' legislative campaign was unsuccessful. Nonetheless, it generated a considerable amount of support from the middle segments of American society. Sympathy for the cause was also forthcoming from the practicing branch of medicine and from the ranks of other professions.[48]

This widespread support for antivivisectionism seems to contradict the historical wisdom that scientific medicine was acquiring cultural authority during the late nineteenth and early twentieth centuries. Why was it that medical science encountered popular opposition and distrust just as it was securing institutional strength and social legitimacy? Richard French suggests that the answer lies in discomfort within the intelligentsia with what its members viewed as the impersonality and ethical insularity of the modern medical profession.[49] As science became the basis for professional standing, notions of character, duty, and morality declined in importance. Those supporting a moderate antivivisectionist position viewed the willingness of doctors to use patients in experiments as an indication that commitment to science was replacing a tradition of medical beneficence. Proponents of scientific medicine endeavored to reground medicine on a foundation of laboratory research. According to French, this involved two fundamental changes: adjusting clinical interventions to conform to the outcome of empirical studies and conceiving of medical practitioners as natural scientists as much as healers. Resistance to these changes emerged from both the rank and file of the medical profession and from segments of the public who viewed them as destructive to the doctor-patient relationship.

The leadership of American medical science mounted a substantial effort to counter the impact of antivivisectionist activism. Their efforts had three components. First, researchers lobbied against legislative restrictions on animal and human experimentation. In the late 1890s, members of the medical establishment—William Welch, dean of the Johns Hopkins Medical School, and William Keen, a prominent surgeon and later president of the American Medical Association (AMA)—appeared before Congress to testify against government regulation. Other scientists—among them Simon Flexner, scientific director of the Rockefeller Institute for Medical Research—spoke before state legislatures in the decades that followed. Second, leaders endeavored to shape the conduct of medical investigators. In 1908, the AMA established the Council for the Defense of Medical Research, under the direction of Walter Cannon, to coordinate efforts in countering antivivisectionist publicity. Cannon endeavored to improve the scientific community's self-policing. Through informal channels, he exhorted scientific laboratories to avoid conducting studies that might inflame critics and urged the editors of medical journals to eliminate language in scientific articles that might rouse antivivisectionist protests. In editorials in the

AMA's journal, he cajoled scientists to secure the consent of their research subjects.[50]

Third, the community articulated its traditions for handling investigatory risks. It was in the context of antivivisectionist attacks that William Osler addressed the moral conduct of human experiments in his 1907 speech to the Congress of American Physicians and Surgeons. Osler insisted that animal tests should precede human trials and that researchers should conduct risky interventions only with the subject's full knowledge and consent. He went on to praise the self-experimentation of past medical researchers. Pamphlets issued by the Council for the Defense of Medical Research also invoked the community's informal morality. Richard M. Pearce, author of *The Charge of "Human Vivisection" as Presented in Antivivisection Literature* (1914), wrote that medical progress required researchers "to make the first tests and experiments on animals and then if found useful and not dangerous to apply them, with every possible safeguard, to the relief of man." This course of action was a "definite ethical principle."[51] Like Osler, Pearce applauded a widespread pattern of self-experimentation among medical investigators.

Publications from the Council for the Defense of Medical Research also included statements of lesser-harm reasoning. Writing in *Vaccination and Its Relation to Animal Experimentation* (1911), Jay F. Schamberg declared that "the danger connected with vaccination is infinitesimal compared with the peril of remaining unvaccinated."[52] Anti-vaccinationists, he continued, enormously exaggerated the risks of vaccination while failing to appreciate the hazards of disease that would result if the public rejected vaccination. Schamberg then offered a narrative that sought to normalize vaccine risks, his wording echoing the text of the British Royal Commission report published a little more than a decade earlier:

> Every human act is accompanied by some measure of danger. When one rides in an elevator, in a railroad car, or even promenades on the sidewalk, he takes a certain definite risk which can be mathematically calculated. While in the aggregate the number of accidents and deaths from each of these cases may be considerable, yet the individual risk is so small that it may be disregarded. It is the same with reference to vaccination.[53]

When articulating their moral traditions, members of the early-twentieth-century scientific community in America borrowed from the formulations of earlier medical researchers. They directed their moral logic toward a variety of audiences: toward the research community in an effort to solidify agreement as to the appropriate conduct of human experiments, and toward the public and the practicing branch of the medical profession in an effort to win support for the techniques and aims of scientific medicine. When addressing outside audiences, the community sought to assure them that human experiments were in the public good and would be conducted appropriately and responsibly.

Self-Experiments and the "Morality of Method"

Thus far I have said relatively little about two features of researcher's traditions for handling investigatory hazards: self-experimentation and the "morality of method"—ideas that link the morality of a risky human intervention to the quality of the investigator's scientific work. Self-experimentation is, in at least one respect, an exception among the components of researchers' informal morality. Its roots lie not in the techniques or logic of modern science but, rather, in the notion of the professional as gentleman. Before the late nineteenth century, the authority of elite practitioners rested, in large measure, on their social class and on the assertion of personal character and honor. As the professions modernized during the late nineteenth and early twentieth centuries, the idea of the medical practitioner as technical expert gained prominence.[54] But older currents of thought remained salient. With self-experimentation, scientists based their claims for the safety of a new procedure—and for the appropriateness of human testing—on personal integrity. The practice was common both before and after the modernization of the profession.[55]

Early-twentieth-century researchers typically refrained from making explicit mention of self-experimentation in their scientific publications.[56] But they had no such reticence when generating professional discourse about moral conduct of clinical experiments. As noted earlier, Osler extolled the heroism of self-experimenting researchers in his 1907 address to the Congress of American Physicians and Surgeons.[57] Researchers readily invoked self-experimentation both when responding to the charge of unjustified human experimentation and when seeking to recruit human research subjects. Pearce's 1914 pamphlet responded to antivivisectionist criticism of human experimentation by pointing to scientists' willingness to go first. In seeking to provide "relief of mankind's suffering from disease," researchers must ultimately proceed to human trials of their innovations. "In these first crucial tests on man, the greatest caution is observed and it is usually the investigator himself who submits to the test. . . . The scientist volunteer is always ready."[58]

Lawrence Altman remarks on the utility of statements about self-experimentation for recruiting human subjects. He quotes a senior scientist at the British Ministry of Health: "It's much easier to get the volunteer's cooperation for a study if you sit by the bedside and say that you have done the same experiment on yourself and are none the worse for it."[59] Interestingly, vaccine researchers tested experimental immunizing agents not only on themselves but also on their children. In the late 1930s and early 1940s, Joseph Stokes Jr. conducted trials with experimental vaccines against influenza and measles at a large number of children's institutions in New Jersey and eastern Pennsylvania. In the course of gaining access to these facilities, Stokes wrote numerous letters to institutional directors and state health officials. When arranging access for experiments with a measles vaccine, Stokes mentioned to several correspondents that he had vaccinated his own daughter with the immunizing agent. These statements were extremely effective in assuaging managers' concerns about the safety of the vaccine.[60] When John Kolmer inaugurated human use of his new live-polio vaccine in 1934, he also conducted tests first on himself and his two children. Later, when responding to inquiries about the appropriateness of his use of research subjects, Kolmer pointed to his prior self-inoculation and to the inoculation of his children.[61] Like self-experimentation, experimenting on one's children demonstrated the researcher's belief in the safety of an immunizing agent and his willingness to face the personal consequences of that conviction.

In contrast to self-experimentation, the "morality of method" is unambiguously rooted in cognitive norms of science. For the most part, this feature of investigators' traditions remained tacit, at least until well into the twentieth century. But the notion that good science is necessary to the moral conduct of human trials was clearly implicit in early lesser-harm formulations. If researchers use unsound methods when conducting a human experiment, no net benefit accrues from its performance, and any risks to which subjects were exposed are unjustified. Furthermore, accurate assessment of the risks and benefits of a prospective intervention rest on the evaluation of empirical findings. If these findings are unreliable or their interpretation faulty, scientists are likely to misjudge the hazards associated with an experimental intervention. Controversy surrounding use of experimental polio vaccines in 1934–35—the subject of chapter 2—illustrates the research community's convictions about the importance of sound scientific work to the morality of proceeding with clinical use of risky medical procedures. So too does the tremendous care Jurin displayed when assessing reports of the outcome of smallpox inoculation. One of D'Alembert's objections to Bernoulli's lesser-harm calculations is further illustration of scientists' insistence on the need for solid evidence: if Bernoulli's data on mortality from natural and inoculated smallpox was inadequate, then practical use of the resulting calculations was morally untenable. Morality of method is also implicit in the debate that surrounded Pasteur's decision to proceed with human use of his rabies vaccine. At issue was whether Pasteur's prior animal tests were sufficient to make valid scientific judgments about the preparation's safety and efficacy for humans.

It was a group of advocates for the reform of medical therapeutics—an intraprofessional movement seeking to bring medical practice into line with research—that made the clearest and most forceful statements of the morality of method. During the early and middle decades of the twentieth century, this movement would redefine the methodological standard used for testing medical therapies. Evaluations based on loosely constructed controls or historical comparisons and on the opinions of trusted colleagues—widely accepted during the early decades of the twentieth century—gave way at midcentury to an insistence on rigorously controlled experiments. In the 1960s, scientific leaders insisted that randomized clinical trials were necessary for the assessment of medical therapies.[62] Proponents of strictly controlled trials made the morality of method explicit. David Rutstein, who in 1970 declared that scientifically sound clinical research was "itself an ethical principle," was a vocal supporter of rigorously controlled trials.[63] He and other proponents of therapeutic reform directed their moral discourse toward the professional community in an effort to win support for the new methodological imperatives.

The advent of rigorously controlled trials would lead to the identification of new moral dilemmas in the conduct of human experiments—for example, whether patients seeking treatment should be forced into randomization. Also, with strictly controlled trials, the line between an experiment and clinical use of an intervention—indistinct in many early vaccine trials—would become less ambiguous. But such developments postdate the endpoint of this volume. For the bulk of the vaccine trials examined in this book, control groups were loosely constituted or nonexistent, and the line between medical experiment and clinical practice was often indistinct.

Moral Rhetoric as a Cultural Resource

Three dynamics regarding expressions of informal morality emerge from the preceding narrative. First, medical innovators' moral logic has been closely tied to their notions about the proper conduct of science. Research communities have grounded their moral traditions both in the reasoning

underlying empirical inquiry and in specific investigatory practices. Sociologists have debated whether the norms of scientific communities are social
or technical in origin.[64] My account suggests that, with the exception of self-
experimentation, medical investigators' traditions for managing hazards
have their roots in the techniques of science.

Second, although researchers' moral logic is largely technical in origin,
the purposes that its expression serves are very often unabashedly social.
Moral traditions have been not only a set of standards for governing use of
risk-laden medical interventions, but also the source of rhetorical strategies.
In each of the major episodes examined in this chapter, the individuals who
voiced researchers' moral logic were constructing a language of persuasion
aimed at establishing or confirming an internal professional consensus.
Quite often, they directed their rhetoric not only toward scientific and medical communities but also toward researchers' lay audiences with the goal of
managing relations with patrons and the broader public.[65]

In the course of inaugurating new clinical techniques, investigators have
repeatedly encountered public alarm over the medical hazards as well as discomfort with the notion of experimenting on humans. Eighteenth-century
scientists confronted resistance to new procedures on the basis of religion
and medical theory. Nineteenth- and early-twentieth-century investigators
faced opposition from organized social movements, activists objecting to
compulsory immunization and to unrestricted animal and human experimentation. These movements—and periodic reports of serious injuries
subsequent to the use of new procedures—stirred public anxieties. The scientific community has given voice to its moral logic in an effort to win acceptance both for new medical interventions and for the experimental methods employed when introducing innovations into clinical practice.

The third dynamic concerns the relationship between early and later
statements of investigatory morality. When scientists have formulated
rhetoric for addressing the distinctive issues facing their professional community, they have borrowed freely from the conceptual and linguistic strategies used by previous researchers. Sociologist Ann Swidler conceives of culture as a toolkit—a repertoire of symbols, images, and rhetorical devices
that social actors can draw upon when constructing strategies for action.[66]
The moral discourse of earlier scientists is a cultural resource readily available to later groups of medical researchers. In the case of one moral tradition, lesser-harm reasoning, scientists' moral discourse became broadly
diffused not only in scientific and professional communities but in public
arenas as well.

2

Negotiating Moral Boundaries:
The Polio Vaccines of 1934–1935

Sociologists consider the problem group, or research network, to be the basic unit in the organization of scientific work. Members of these networks address common questions, share research materials, and exchange information on research techniques. They evaluate one another's findings and arrive at agreements as to what constitutes scientific truth.[1] Problem groups are also bearers and adjudicators of moral traditions for handling investigatory risk. Their assessments of research findings are vital to applications of lesser-harm reasoning. Estimates of the hazards and benefits of a medical intervention rest on the interpretation of existing empirical findings, and research networks are a primary location for such interpretations. Problem groups collectively evaluate evidence concerning the risks and benefits of proposed interventions and, in part on that basis, make judgments about the acceptability of human experiments.

In this chapter, I examine a case in which a research network acted to stop the use of vaccines that it deemed too hazardous. In July of 1934, two groups of American researchers, each with its own immunizing agent, began human vaccinations against poliomyelitis. From the outset, members of the community of virus researchers had questions about the vaccines' safety and efficacy. Uncertainties surrounded the assessment of empirical evidence relevant to the vaccines' risks and benefits. Scientists were struggling to arrive at a consensus about the preparations' dangers and merits when they received reports that a number of vaccine recipients had contracted paralytic polio. Several died. The vaccines' initiators insisted that the affected children had been exposed to polio prior to immunization. But their colleagues were alarmed by the deaths and doubtful of the validity of the experimenters' claims. Key members of the problem group repudiated the immunizing agents and advised the sponsor of one vaccine to withdraw its funding. By December 1935, human use of the preparations had ceased.

Analysis of the 1934–35 polio-vaccine controversy clarifies the ways that the technical culture of science comes to play in deliberations over the morality of human experiments. When interpreting evidence relevant to hazards and benefits, scientists base their evaluations on what some scholars have called "local knowledge": hands-on familiarity with the techniques and materials used in producing empirical findings.[2] Clifford Geertz remarks that "the shapes of knowledge are . . . ineluctably local, indivisible from their instruments and their encasements."[3] Local knowledge relevant to evaluations of experimental risks and benefits includes familiarity with cell lines and laboratory procedures as well as with the reputations of the scientists conducting the research. In deliberations over the acceptability of human application of a laboratory intervention, technical issues have moral stature.

My account also points to the importance that research networks place on the legitimacy of human interventions to outside audiences. Scientists know they must operate within the bounds of public tolerance for investigatory risk. Assessments of hazards and benefits are often both uncertain and contested. Disagreements about the dangers of one of the two 1935 polio vaccines were never fully resolved. Some viewed its risks as low when compared to the benefits of a workable intervention against polio. But deaths attributable to the other vaccine had occurred, and one prominent scientist privately invoked the specter of a lay investigation of vaccine injuries. Research leaders took action to prevent the possibility of further human harm, to forestall outside inquiries, and to protect public trust in future immunizing agents.

My narrative sheds light on the character of an early-twentieth-century problem group and its capacity for moral oversight. Research networks are carriers of both an indigenous morality and the expertise crucial for assessing experimental risks and benefits. But their ability to constrain the behavior of members has limits. As is the case with other loosely constituted groups, the pressures that a research network exerts on its members are informal ones. The principal means for social control is granting and withholding prestige. Scientists conform to group norms to maintain the esteem of their colleagues. Researchers who fail to conform may find themselves ostracized or treated as marginal.[4] But when such informal pressures fail to work, research networks are poorly equipped to impose more coercive controls. Key members of the polio-research community in 1935 did take coercive action. But the circumstances were unusual. Professional leaders moved only when the situation had become extreme, and their success was due in large measure to their influence with the organizational sponsor of one of the vaccines.

American Polio Researchers in the Early Twentieth Century

By the early 1930s, well over a hundred American investigators had tried their hand at laboratory experiments with poliovirus.[5] Most had research agendas that included problems other than poliomyelitis or focused on the virus for a circumscribed time period. These scientists worked in a variety of settings: medical schools, public health laboratories, research institutes, and at the federal Hygienic Laboratory—renamed the National Institute of Health (NIH) in 1930. Their correspondence reveals that early polio researchers participated in colleague networks similar to those operating among present-day medical investigators. They exchanged virus specimens, details about their laboratory procedures, and informal reports of ongoing experiments. In addition to written communications, they met at special sessions on poliomyelitis at research conferences and at committees on clinical aspects of the disease sponsored by public health and voluntary agencies.

A combination of public health, scientific, and institutional factors contributed to the emergence of polio studies as an arena of laboratory research. Concern with polio as a health problem was central. Epidemics of paralytic poliomyelitis, also known as infantile paralysis, were recurrent in America beginning in the final decade of the nineteenth century. Rates of the disease were low relative to other epidemic illnesses, even during polio outbreaks. But the unpredictability of polio's appearance and clinical outcome generated tremendous anxiety. Polio could result in either death or permanent, disabling paralysis. While the disease sometimes sickened young adults, its victims were most often infants and children.[6]

Contemporary medicine offered no means for altering the clinical course of poliomyelitis or for preventing new cases. Two immunizing agents would become widely available just after midcentury—the Salk vaccine during the mid-1950s and the Sabin vaccine in the early 1960s. Until then, isolation and quarantine were the principal tools available for controlling polio's spread. Health officials began using quarantine to the fullest during a 1916 epidemic in the northeastern United States that generated 27,000 cases—9,000 in

New York City alone. As late as the early 1950s, it was typical for summer camps and swimming pools to close during polio epidemics. Fear of the disease led many parents to confine healthy youngsters to the house during outbreaks and to remove children from locations with ongoing cases. Through the 1950s, commentators depicted polio as the most dreaded disease of childhood.[7]

Scientific and institutional developments also fostered the growth of polio research. On the scientific side were the results of early experimental studies. In 1908, the Viennese researcher Karl Landsteiner succeeded in infecting monkeys with human poliomyelitis. During the following year, several research groups identified the disease-causing agent as a filterable virus. By the end of 1909, scientists in Austria, Germany, France, and America had accomplished both human-to-monkey and monkey-to-monkey transfers of paralytic polio. Simon Flexner, scientific director of the Rockefeller Institute for Medical Research in New York City, headed the first group to report serial transfers.[8] At that time, scientists were unable to keep viruses alive outside living organisms. The practical implication of serial transfers of polio in monkeys was that researchers could study the experimental disease, and measures to prevent it, in the laboratory.

On the institutional side was the creation of full-time appointments for researchers at American medical schools and other professional organizations during the early twentieth century. New career tracks facilitated the overall growth of medical science.[9] Funding targeted for studies of polio encouraged members of the growing cadre of medical scientists to direct their efforts toward infantile paralysis. Charitable organizations responded to early polio outbreaks by making support available for experimental studies of the disease. The Rockefeller Foundation—administratively distinct from the Rockefeller Institute—began to support polio research during the 1916 epidemic. The New York City philanthropist Jeremiah Milbank allocated a quarter million dollars for experimental work on polio during the late 1920s. In the mid-1930s, the President's Birthday Ball Commission (PBBC), a charity established by friends of Franklin D. Roosevelt—whose paralytic illness was diagnosed as polio—dispensed an equally large pool of funds for laboratory studies on poliomyelitis. These were substantial sums of money for that period. Milbank's grantees produced eighty scientific papers in a period of four years. PBBC funds supported the work of sixteen groups of laboratory investigators.[10]

Early polio researchers directed their efforts toward a number of questions. They aimed a good deal of their work toward better understanding of the nature of poliomyelitis and improving experimental tools for studying it. Scientists explored the physiology of the poliomyelitis infection and the mechanisms of its transmission. They applied techniques—crude by today's standards—for identifying the presence of antibodies to poliovirus. They repeatedly tried to infect animals other than primates with polio so that further experimental studies could be conducted with animals that were easier to obtain and handle in the laboratory. Curative and preventive measures were never far from their sights. In an effort to develop a treatment for infantile paralysis, researchers extracted serum from animals and humans recovering from the disease in the hopes that these preparations would impart passive immunity. Human testing of serum preparations began in earnest during the 1916 epidemic and continued through the early 1930s. Meanwhile, researchers worked toward achieving their ultimate goal: a safe and effective polio vaccine.[11]

After the experimental breakthroughs of the late 1910s, Flexner and other polio investigators were optimistic that laboratory research would quickly yield measures for preventing and treating paralytic polio. But problems encountered in developing immunizing agents would remain unresolved for decades. Serum treatment of poliomyelitis never proved to be effective, and attempts at producing a polio vaccine were repeatedly unsuccessful. Scientists developed both attenuated live-virus and killed-virus vaccines. They tried a wide array of techniques for altering the poliovirus. But their efforts were to no avail. Killed-virus preparations were unreliable in producing immunity. Some live-virus preparations generated immunity but also caused paralytic polio in a portion of experimental animals.[12] Attempts at vaccine development were ongoing in the early 1930s, but few polio researchers viewed the human testing of a laboratory-generated immunizing agent to be on the immediate horizon.

Moral Traditions Observed

Polio investigators fully embraced the informal morality of the broader medical-research community. When addressing possible human use of polio vaccines, they observed the expectations identified earlier as core features of scientists' traditions for handling experimental hazards. Polio researchers appealed to a risk-benefit calculus when considering human use of a vaccine. They would engage in self-experimentation before using the vaccine on other human recipients. They derided research they viewed as scientifically unsound. They insisted that animal experiments precede human trials. They refrained from human testing when they judged the hazards to be too great and halted use of preparations whose risk they had underestimated. Indeed, with the exception of the two vaccines employed briefly in 1934–35, scientists observed a moratorium against the human testing of polio vaccines through the first half of the twentieth century.[13]

Simon Flexner spearheaded the moratorium among American researchers shortly after his success with serial transfers of poliovirus. Flexner was at the center of the American polio-research community during the 1910s and 1920s. He supplied poliovirus to many of the early generations of researchers and kept abreast of their subsequent work. As scientific director of the prestigious Rockefeller Institute and internationally recognized for his own research, Flexner was well positioned to affect the behavior of other investigators. Among his aims was to ensure that no researcher began human use of a polio vaccine until the problems with immunizing agents were solved with animals. Toward this end, Flexner included warnings against human vaccinations in his early publications. In a 1910 article he insisted, "At present, the experimental basis is entirely inadequate to justify the attempt to induce active immunity as a protective measure in human beings."[14] His cautionary remarks extended not only to the testing of vaccines but to the use of immune sera as well:

> Serum treatment of poliomyelitis must at the present time be regarded as strictly in the experimental state, and it cannot be predicted how soon or whether ever at all such a form of specific treatment of the disease will be applicable to the spontaneous epidemic disease in human beings.[15]

Flexner went beyond published statements by including warnings against human inoculations in his correspondence with contemporary researchers. In November of 1911, Hans Zinsser, then an associate professor of bacteriology at Stanford University, wrote to Flexner about injecting monkeys with spinal-cord tissue from several deceased patients suspected to have had poliomyelitis. Zinsser was also injecting rabbits with the spinal-cord tissue. Flexner anticipated where Zinsser's efforts might be heading:

> I feel I should warn you against the inoculation of human beings with poliomyelitis virus. It is a very uncertain organism, even in monkeys. I have referred to the matter in one of the reprints to warn against any vaccination of the sort. Besides, I do not believe that a few cases [of polio] in any community is grounds for the vaccination of the well.[16]

Flexner further elaborated his position in a letter sent a week later:

> [My previous letter] explains my views concerning the question of vaccina-
> tion for poliomyelitis. I am also inclined to discourage you from the treat-
> ment of human beings with the rabbit serum until you have tried the
> serum on the experimental disease in monkeys. Now that the disease is
> subject to experimental tests of therapeutic agents it seems to me quite
> wrong to make any hypothetical tests on human beings, because, as I view
> it, you may not only do no good but you run the risk of doing actual harm.[17]

Zinsser responded: "I am heeding your advice regarding the caution to be
exercised in applying any experimental treatment to human beings and
shall certainly do nothing of the sort should other cases arise."[18]

The delay in human testing of immune sera was temporary. As already
noted, therapeutic use of polio serum became common during the 1916 epidemic. But the moratorium on human use of polio vaccines held. In the late
1920s and early 1930s, the balance of opinion about active immunization
against infantile paralysis was much as it had been two decades earlier. Researchers continued to find killed-virus preparations ineffective and live-
virus vaccines both unreliable and unsafe. With preparations that showed
promise for generating immunity, "now and again a treated monkey suc-
cumb[ed] to the disease as a result of the inoculations."[19] Investigators restated the consensus in scientific papers and in a 1932 review of the polio-
research field published by the Milbank-sponsored International Committee for the Study of Infantile Paralysis.[20]

Lesser-harm reasoning was a prominent feature of discussions of polio-
vaccine use. To be acceptable for human application, the hazards of the immunizing agent had to be lower than the risks of the natural disease. With
infantile paralysis, this implied a very safe vaccine, for despite public fear of
the disease, incidence of paralytic polio was actually quite low. The authors
of the Milbank Committee report questioned whether human use of polio
vaccines would ever be prevalent: "In view of the low morbidity rate of poliomyelitis, widespread active immunization of human beings would probably never be attempted, even if a method of proved success were available."
They did leave open the possibility of vaccination when polio outbreaks were
occurring: "During epidemic periods . . . any means that offers a possibility
of controlling the spread, would be eagerly sought."[21]

Perhaps the clearest articulation of lesser-harm logic occurred in the
aftermath of the polio-vaccine controversy. Sidney Kramer, a researcher

at the Long Island College of Medicine—later SUNY Downstate Medical Center—discussed the acceptability of human use of immunizing agents against poliomyelitis. Kramer developed his own polio vaccine during the 1930s but refrained from proceeding with human trials. His remarks were a commentary on the two recently discredited polio vaccines:

> Paralytic poliomyelitis remains a comparatively uncommon disease. . . . Were we dealing with a more common disease, an immunizing agent of high effectiveness, even though it occasionally resulted in the accidental production of the disease, might still be the means of protecting a great many individuals. In the case of a rare disease like poliomyelitis, one such accident in several hundred, or even several thousand, would approach the incidence of the [natural] disease and thus negate any value that would accrue.[22]

James Leake, a researcher and medical officer at the U.S. Public Health Service, endorsed Kramer's logic but argued for a higher standard of safety. Leake insisted that the incidence of paralytic polio in the general population was one in ten thousand individuals.[23] The implication of Leake's point was clear. One death or serious injury among ten thousand polio-vaccine recipients was not safe enough.

Two Short-Lived Vaccines

The informal moratorium on human testing of vaccines against poliomyelitis ended in July of 1934 when two different groups of researchers began clinical trials.[24] William Park and Maurice Brodie at the New York City Public Health Department Laboratory introduced one of the preparations. The Health Department Laboratory had been producing immunizing agents since the 1890s, when it had initiated distribution of diphtheria antitoxin. Park had been the laboratory's director for nearly forty years and had national standing in both the medical-research and public health communities. In 1933, Park hired Brodie, a promising young medical investigator from McGill University, to pursue the development of a polio vaccine. Park secured funding for Brodie's work from the New York Foundation, the Rockefeller Foundation, and beginning in 1935, the PBBC.

John Kolmer developed and initiated use of the other vaccine. Kolmer headed an entrepreneurial research institute in Philadelphia called the Institute for Cutaneous Medicine (ICM), which had started out as an independent laboratory. Its founders had supplied Salvarsan—a brand of arsphenamine, used in the treatment of syphilis—to the U.S. Army during World War I. At the war's end, they used their considerable earnings to endow a not-for-profit corporation that supported medical research. Kolmer was prominent in the Philadelphia medical community and, in the mid-1930s, held an appointment at Temple University Medical School. A fund for research on neurology at Temple provided some support for Kolmer's polio-vaccine studies.[25]

The Brodie and Kolmer vaccines had similarities to the immunizing agents that Jonas Salk and Albert Sabin would introduce two decades later. Brodie's preparation, like Salk's, was a killed-virus vaccine inactivated by treatment with formalin, a formaldehyde solution. Kolmer described his preparation—as Sabin would his—as an attenuated live-virus vaccine. Kolmer reported that he had weakened the poliovirus by exposing it to the chemical sodium ricineolate. Sabin attenuated his viruses by a number of procedures, including serial passage through mice—a technique not yet developed in the 1930s. Although the polio vaccines of the 1930s and the 1950s were similar in some respects, at least three crucial differences in underlying science divided them. First, consistent with contemporary scientific wisdom, Brodie and Kolmer assumed the existence of only one strain of poliovirus. By the 1950s, researchers had identified three antigenetically distinct strains of poliovirus. Salk and Sabin included all three in their immunizing agents. Second, pre–World War II scientists had no way to grow poliovirus outside a living host and no animal hosts other than primates. Kolmer and Brodie prepared their vaccines directly from the spinal-cord tissue of polio-infected monkeys. Salk and Sabin had access to techniques for growing poliovirus in tissue-culture media developed during the late 1940s. The resulting vaccines were much cleaner preparations and less likely to generate allergic reactions.[26] Third, early researchers held what were later understood to be inaccurate notions about the physiology of poliomyelitis and its means of transmission. Flexner and his contemporaries believed that polio started as a respiratory infection, invading the host through the nose and proceeding from there to the central nervous system. By midcentury, scientists had discovered that poliovirus enters and exits the body through the gastrointestinal route. In part for this reason, Sabin administered his live-virus vaccine orally. Kolmer administered his preparation by injection, a method that—in hindsight—is likely to be both less effective and ultimately more dangerous.

Both Brodie and Kolmer followed a sequence then customary in the clinical testing of new immunizing agents: animal experiments, self-experiments, small-scale human testing to assess safety, followed by larger-scale human trials to evaluate efficacy. Kolmer initially tried his preparation on forty-two monkeys, Brodie on twenty. The first publications reporting use of the vaccines in monkeys appeared in June of 1934.[27] Both men began self-experimentation during that summer. Kolmer and his assistant tried the vaccine on themselves, on Kolmer's two children (ages eleven and fifteen), and then on twenty-three additional youngsters. Brodie and Park administered their vaccine to six volunteers at the New York City Health Department and then to twelve children in a New York City asylum. By the time the trials ended, Kolmer reported that more than 10,700 individuals had received his vaccine agent. Park and Brodie claimed another 10,000 recipients.[28] Whether these claims were well grounded or not, it is clear that the great bulk of vaccinated individuals received inoculations not from Kolmer, Brodie, or their laboratories, but rather from private medical practices or public health agencies that had obtained supplies of vaccine from one of the research teams. In 1935, NIH's division of biologicals licensed laboratories that manufactured vaccines sold across state lines, but no agency regulated the use of unlicensed immunizing agents.[29] Furthermore, the line between a vaccine experiment and clinical use of an unapproved immunizing agent was indistinct. The practice of distributing newly developed vaccines to physicians and public health agencies for "experimental use" meant that researchers sometimes lacked accurate information about performance of their own immunizing agents, and this contributed to difficulties evaluating safety and efficacy.

From today's standpoint, the course of Brodie's and Kolmer's research is remarkable for the small number of animal experiments they conducted and the rapidity with which they proceeded to human testing. John Paul suggests that competition between the two investigators fueled a rush into human trials.[30] Their dependence on primates as laboratory animals may also provide a partial explanation for the team's quick move to human trials. Monkeys were the staple of laboratory research on polio. Researchers used them to create their immunizing agents—at Park's laboratory, one sacrificed monkey produced ten doses of vaccine. Monkeys served as the animal subjects for tests of vaccine safety and efficacy. In addition, researchers sacrificed animals when assessing the antibody levels of human recipients of the vaccine. Tests for antibodies before and after vaccination provided an indication of vaccine efficacy in the absence of the subjects' known exposure to natural polio.[31] But monkeys and other primates were scarce, expensive to purchase, and difficult to maintain in laboratory settings. Shortages of monkeys were a continual problem for polio researchers in the 1930s, and scientists complained that the limited supply inhibited research.[32]

In addition to competition between research groups and a shortage of monkeys, other factors may also have contributed to the breakdown of the polio-vaccine moratorium. Confidence in the efficacy of convalescent-serum treatment for infantile paralysis was fading. Clinical studies published in the early 1930s showed that serum treatment was of no benefit. Meanwhile, anxiety about recurrent outbreaks of polio gave urgency to the work of finding a vaccine. The availability of funding for polio-vaccine research was encouraging the development of experimental immunizing agents. Changes in the colleague network were occurring as well. With Flexner's impending retirement as scientific director of the Rockefeller Institute effective October 1935, and a widening range of researchers entering the field, power within the network was less highly centralized than it had been earlier. Flexner had shaped scientific thinking about polio for twenty-five years. Some within the expanding circle of polio virologists were questioning the conventional wisdom established by senior researchers.[33] Whatever the precise combination of reasons, the moratorium on human testing of polio vaccines ended for a short time midway through 1934.

Local Knowledge

Reports that two investigators had begun human use of polio vaccines created a stir in the research community. If either Brodie or Kolmer had indeed created a safe and effective vaccine, it represented a tremendous breakthrough for the fields of virology and public health. However, many established scientists were skeptical of the claims Kolmer and Brodie were making for their vaccines. Since the advent of an animal model for polio in 1909, many well-respected researchers had tried and failed to develop a vaccine that reliably generated immunity to polio without infecting some experimental animals with the disease. If Kolmer's and Brodie's statements were to be believed, they had quickly solved problems that had stumped good investigators for years. It remained to be seen whether their reported successes were real or illusory.

Kolmer and Brodie broke with professional protocol by issuing press releases about their human inoculations in September of 1934, before they had presented their findings to the scientific community.[34] They delivered professional addresses and published papers only later that fall.[35] In the months that followed, polio researchers struggled to assess the new vaccines. Debates took place not only between the vaccine innovators and their critics but also among members of the research community more generally. Central figures in the controversy included scientists at the Rockefeller In-

stitute (Simon Flexner, Thomas Rivers, and Peter Olitsky), researchers at
NIH and the broader Public Health Service (George McCoy, James Leake,
and Charles Armstrong), and scientific advisors to the PBBC (particularly
Paul de Kruif, George McCoy, and later, Thomas Rivers). Others playing an
important role included Lloyd Aycock at Harvard, Sidney Kramer at Long Island Medical College, and Karl Meyer, who was affiliated with both the University of California at San Francisco and the Hooper Institute. While some
aspects of the debate took place in journal articles and at professional sym-
posia, the most consequential interactions occurred in informal communications among members of the research community.

Three features of scientists' discussions of the new vaccines are especially noteworthy. First, arguments during the heat of the controversy placed
less emphasis on the logic of lesser harms than on the science of vaccine development. Questions about risks and benefits quickly resolved into questions about the soundness of Kolmer's and Brodie's scientific claims and the
interpretation of empirical evidence: Were the preparations sufficiently attenuated to avoid generating paralytic polio in even a tiny portion of vaccine
recipients? Would the vaccines really provide immunity against future exposures to poliomyelitis? Answers to questions about the vaccines' hazards
and merits rested on judgments about the meaning of empirical evidence. It
was evaluation of this evidence, contested among members of the research
community, that was at issue during the polio-vaccine controversy.

Second, the assuredness conveyed in statements about lesser harms
made before and after the vaccines' use gave way to uncertainty about the
preparations' efficacy and safety. Twenty years of laboratory studies of polio
made investigators skeptical of the vaccine innovators' claims for their immunizing agents. Again, the research community was simply unsure about
whether Kolmer's and Brodie's experimental techniques were sound or
their interpretations of data accurate. Third, consistent with the notion of local knowledge, researchers based their evaluation of colleagues' research
findings on their own familiarity with both laboratory techniques and the
behavior of viruses and on their judgments about the investigatory skills of
scientists at other laboratories.

Early evaluations of Kolmer's work were unfavorable. Kolmer was a pe-
ripheral figure in the polio-research community. Those within it who knew
him thought Kolmer was, at best, inexperienced with poliovirus. In 1932, a
year and a half before starting human tests of his vaccine, Kolmer had written to Simon Flexner requesting a specimen of polio and asking basic questions about laboratory methods for handling the virus.[36] Flexner had forwarded a specimen of virus but also sent Kolmer a list of readings and

suggested that, if Kolmer had not worked with viruses before, he would do better to begin with one less difficult than polio.[37] Flexner later found little reason to revise his assessment of either Kolmer's investigatory skill or the dangers of live-polio vaccines. Kolmer failed to provide experienced polio researchers with a convincing account of why his vaccine should be considered safe for human use. His claims were insufficient to override their own experience in the laboratory as well as an existing body of research. Others shared Flexner's opinion about Kolmer's preparation. Among them was George McCoy, director of NIH and chairman of the PBBC's Medical Advisory Committee. While equivocal about Kolmer's vaccine in public statements, McCoy made his sentiments known privately. On the advice of its scientific advisors, the PBBC provided funding for Park and Brodie's vaccine early in 1935, but not for Kolmer's. Paul de Kruif, secretary to the PBBC, described McCoy's position on the matter in a letter to Jeremiah Milbank, the commission's vice chairman: "McCoy is absolutely not in favor of our doing anything about the Kolmer project. For the reason that he does not believe the injection of living and still infectious virus into children is justified."[38]

Researchers' concerns about Brodie's vaccine had less to do with safety than efficacy. Still, some scientists were uncomfortable with Brodie's work. They complained that he had failed to document his laboratory methods fully and that he made inconsistent statements about his vaccine. Rivers reviewed Brodie's work for the Rockefeller Foundation, one of Brodie's funders. In a memo to Foundation personnel, Rivers declared that Brodie "never tells exactly the same story. Once he stated that the virus is dead, but in Chicago he admitted that some of the virus might and probably was alive. I think he should get very accurate data on the state of the virus in his vaccine."[39]

In March of 1935, Brodie submitted a paper, "Active Immunization of Children against Poliomyelitis," to the *Journal of Experimental Medicine*. Brodie had published a brief account of his initial human tests of polio vaccine in November of 1934. But as yet, no full description of the human trials had appeared in a scientific publication. Peyton Rous, a Rockefeller Institute researcher and editor of the journal, forwarded Brodie's paper to Flexner for review. Flexner responded that he deplored Brodie's "slapdash way of working." Flexner continued excitedly: "I cannot understand Brodie's figure for effective doses; minute details are required here. I have never secured such precise figures, nor has anyone else, with poliomyelitis virus—a deceptive substance."[40] At issue was whether Brodie was really able to "titrate accurately and regularly 1 minimum completely paralyzing dose [for monkeys] of virus," because he was preparing doses of the human vaccine on the basis of that measurement.[41] Flexner told Rous that he favored publication of the paper if Brodie provided proper documentation. Flexner then wrote to Brodie, inviting the younger scientist to his office for a chat.[42] Brodie's paper did not subsequently appear in the *Journal of Experimental Medicine*.

Charles Armstrong, who oversaw research on poliomyelitis at NIH and worked with McCoy, also had questions about Brodie's procedures. De Kruif at the PBBC noted that Armstrong had found "some discrepancies" in Brodie's published accounts. De Kruif urged that Park and Brodie meet with NIH scientists to "iron out" problems.[43] McCoy would remain skeptical about the efficacy of Brodie's vaccine, but he did support PBBC funding for research to evaluate its merits.[44]

While highly critical of claims by Kolmer and Brodie in private communications, researchers were more circumspect when speaking on the record. Park, a well-respected vaccine researcher for forty years, insisted Brodie's work was sound—and Park's word carried weight. Not everyone was convinced that use of Kolmer's vaccine was a bad idea. Morris Fishbein, editor of the *Journal of the American Medical Association (JAMA)* and widely regarded as a spokesman for the practicing branch of the profession, made public statements about the "remarkable progress" Kolmer had made.[45] There was also the practical side of the poliomyelitis problem to consider. American parents dreaded polio and were eager to try even untested methods to protect their children.[46] Press coverage of the vaccines was raising public expectations that an effective intervention against paralytic polio was at hand. In February of 1935, the *New York Times* reported that use of Brodie's vaccine had been a success in California where it had been used in a polio epidemic during the summer of 1934.[47] The research community's public position was that the Kolmer and Brodie preparations were experimental vaccines whose safety and efficacy were yet to be determined. Scientists who faulted Kolmer or Brodie for failing to produce compelling evidence were going to be held to their own standards.

Uncertainties Prevail

During the first half of the twentieth century, no federal agency controlled use of experimental immunizing agents. NIH's charge did include licensing laboratories that produced commercially available vaccines and sera. But regulating the investigational use of immunizing agents—use not involving sale—fell outside its legal mandate. When federal officials commented on the polio vaccines, it was to emphasize their experimental status. In February of 1935, when publicity about the vaccines was at a peak, the U.S. surgeon general, Hugh S. Cummings, prepared a statement about the immunizing agents:

> Numerous inquiries have reached me regarding the advisability of the inoculation of children against poliomyelitis. This is a personal matter, to be determined according to the circumstances, but several considerations should be borne in mind. None of the methods have been proved to be efficacious and absolutely harmless. Some thousand inoculations must be made under conditions such that the results will be definitely known before this proof is available. For my own family, I should want assurance of a real advantage, in protection from a definite hazard, or in knowledge commensurate to the risk, before poliomyelitis inoculation is made.[48]

In August 1935, McCoy restated the stance of the U.S. Public Health Service, NIH's parent agency:

> The position of the Service is that neither the Kolmer nor the Park-Brodie vaccine is of proven value and both are to be used only experimentally in a view to determining their field of usefulness, if any. I personally, would not give either vaccine to children in the expectation of preventing poliomyelitis. I would give it to them as an experiment to determine whether or not the vaccine is effective.[49]

Although in his official capacity as head of NIH, McCoy routinely refrained from taking sides in scientific controversies, he was, as noted earlier, less guarded in his role as a member of the PBBC's scientific advisory board, supporting funding for Brodie's vaccine but not for Kolmer's.[50]

Faced with uncertainty about the risks and benefits of the polio vaccines, the research community sought independent empirical evidence bearing on the immunizing agents' safety and efficacy. To this end, scientists initiated both laboratory experiments and field trials. Investigators at three institutions sought to replicate Kolmer's and Brodie's animal studies: Edwin Schultz at Stanford University, Sidney Kramer at Long Island Medical College, and Peter Olitsky and Herald Cox at the Rockefeller Institute. According to Rivers, Olitsky and Cox were working under Flexner's direction.[51] Meanwhile, the Public Health Service made plans to conduct a controlled field trial of Brodie's vaccine. The agency sent Alexander Gilliam and Robert Onstott to North Carolina during the summer of 1935 to evaluate vaccine effectiveness in locations where epidemic polio was anticipated. Leake oversaw their work. Lloyd Aycock from Harvard collaborated by examining polio antibodies in vaccinated and unvaccinated subjects. Meanwhile, Park arranged for further use of Brodie's vaccine in southern California where epidemic conditions continued during the spring and summer of 1935.

By early summer of 1935, the outcome of animal replication studies was circulating among polio researchers. The three groups conducting animal studies found that neither Kolmer's nor Brodie's vaccine protected monkeys against later exposure to unmodified poliovirus. In July, Rivers recounted the outcome of Schultz's and Olitsky's studies in response to an inquiry. Rivers wrote that Schultz had "repeated Brodie's work in monkeys and found some antibodies in the serum of vaccinated animals, but no increased resistance to infection." Olitsky, he continued, "repeated Brodie's work and cannot demonstrate an increased resistance to infection in spite of the development of a few humoral antibodies. . . . Monkeys vaccinated according to Kolmer's method are little if any better protected than those handled according to Brodie's technique."[52] Meanwhile, Kramer had reported to the Rockefeller Foundation in July that his work showed Brodie's vaccine to be "totally ineffective in the protection of monkeys."[53] In addition, Rivers had received word from Brodie that "the serum content of the antibodies for polio virus in the children vaccinated 8 months ago has gradually fallen and is now approaching the level at which it was before vaccination."[54]

But even though these results further undermined confidence in Brodie's and Kolmer's claims, some scientists did not rule out the possibility that the vaccines might prove effective for immunizing humans. As Rivers commented, "There is very little experimental evidence . . . to show that the vaccines are efficient. Still, one does not know how much protection a human being needs to stop the disease under natural conditions. Consequently, I am not too dogmatic in my statements."[55]

Nor did the summer field studies produce definitive results. Public Health Service researchers sought to conduct a clinical trial with randomly assigned experimental and control groups. "So far as we are aware," Gilliam and Onstott wrote, "no such rigidly controlled clinical study has been undertaken to evaluate this, or any other vaccine."[56] Approximately 450 children were in the experimental group. But no cases of polio occurred among either the vaccinated or unvaccinated children included in the trial. Meanwhile, Aycock and Hudson found that differences in the presence of antibodies between immunized and unimmunized individuals were statistically insignificant.[57] Investigators were facing strategic and technical difficulties that often arise in the conduct of vaccine field trials. A number of realities made polio-vaccine outcome studies particularly difficult: many children had natural immunity to infantile paralysis; the incidence of the disease was low; the course of epidemics was difficult to predict; and even an effective vaccine would not trigger immunity in all recipients. Researchers agreed about the implications of their initial attempts at field testing: a very large clinical study would be needed to generate statistically significant results regarding the effectiveness of a polio vaccine.[58]

Meanwhile, McCoy was concerned about serious allergic reactions to the immunizing agents. In an August memorandum to the assistant surgeon general, McCoy wrote, "It is not possible to say definitely that either [vaccine] is harmless. Possibly the introduction of the amount of nerve tissue required may not be entirely free of risk."[59] McCoy had first voiced such concerns to the PBBC in June of 1935.[60] Experience with clinical use of the vaccine did not allay his fears. John Kessel, who oversaw the administration of the vaccines to health care professionals at Los Angeles County Hospital, reported "a number of severe constitutional reactions, nine among those receiving the Brodie vaccine and five among those receiving the Kolmer vaccine."[61] Gilliam and Onstott also reported "alarming reactions" among vaccine recipients in North Carolina.[62] Park pressed McCoy in early September about the likelihood of further PBBC funding for the production of Brodie's vaccine. McCoy responded, "I am so uncertain about the value of the vaccine in practical application and so apprehensive of some accident occurring, that as you see, I am quite lukewarm on the whole subject."[63]

Drawing Moral Boundaries

The turning point for the vaccines' use came in the fall of 1935. It was then that researchers learned that children inoculated with Kolmer's vaccine had contracted polio. In September, New Jersey public health officials sent Brodie reports of four cases of paralytic polio—three of them fatal—among children vaccinated with Kolmer's preparation. These children had received immunizations one or two weeks before the onset of their illnesses. Brodie forwarded the reports to Rivers, who had them notarized on October 4. Additional cases surfaced in the weeks that followed. By the time the dust settled, Kolmer had acknowledged ten cases of paralytic polio and five deaths among children inoculated with his vaccine—but he denied that the vaccine was responsible.[64] Researchers had predicted that a live-virus preparation like Kolmer's might generate polio among a portion of recipients. They now concluded that their fears had been realized.

Scientists at the Rockefeller Institute moved quickly to repudiate the continued use of Kolmer's vaccine. On October 5, Flexner wrote to Rivers to inform him that "because of the exigencies of the practical situation," he had arranged for a note to appear in *Science*.[65] Flexner's brief paper, published November 1, took issue with Kolmer's claims concerning the safety of his vaccine. Referring in part to Olitsky and Cox's forthcoming findings, Flexner insisted that no known method for attenuating live poliovirus rendered it both effective and safe for human use. Meanwhile, Rivers had agreed to address an October 8 session on the polio vaccines at the American Public Health Association (APHA) meetings in Milwaukee at which Brodie and Kolmer were also presenting papers. Rivers later remarked that his colleagues had sent him to Milwaukee to act as the "hatchet man."[66] His comments on Kolmer's vaccine anticipated Flexner's forthcoming *Science* article. Rivers made it clear that, in the view of the scientific community, Kolmer had provided no empirical evidence to support the contention that his vaccine was safe for human use. The onus was on Kolmer to do so, given the mortality from post-vaccination polio, the time of onset of the illnesses, and the location of the first signs of paralysis—proximal to the site of immunization. Rivers, who had been appointed to the PBBC's scientific advisory board and was knowledgeable about activities at Park's laboratory, also discussed the Park-Brodie preparation. He pointed out that Brodie had been shortening the duration of formalin treatment to improve the vaccine's efficacy, and he advised that further curtailment of treatment might render the vaccine unsafe. Nonetheless, Rivers favored continued research on the preparation's effectiveness and proposed a field trial of 100,000 subjects.[67]

Despite what others viewed as overwhelming evidence to the contrary, Kolmer continued to maintain that his vaccine was safe. Kolmer might have avoided open condemnation had he withdrawn his vaccine at this time. Instead, he insisted that the cases of polio among immunized children were unrelated to the vaccine. In his view, the children had been exposed to polio before immunization and the vaccinations had occurred too late to stop clinical manifestation of the disease.[68]

At this point, the Public Health Service sought a ruling from government attorneys as to whether Kolmer was violating the law by distributing his immunizing agent. NIH had not licensed Kolmer's laboratory. Leake, who had initiated the inquiry, submitted the request to lawyers at the Treasury Department in which the Public Health Service was housed. A memo dated October 23 indicates that the Treasury Department's general counsel found the distribution of Kolmer's vaccine to be legal. As discussed earlier, NIH jurisdiction was limited to laboratories that produced vaccines and other biological materials for commercial sale. But Kolmer was not selling his preparation. Ordering Kolmer to stop dispensing it free of charge was not within the Public Health Service's regulatory mandate.[69]

On November 19, the southern branch of the APHA, meeting in St. Louis, held a special session on poliomyelitis. Kolmer presented a paper addressing the ten cases of post-vaccination polio. Many of the principal researchers in the field were in attendance. Kolmer again proclaimed his vaccine to be safe, insisting that infected children had contracted polio prior to vaccination. In a later interview, Rivers describes what happened at the end of Kolmer's address:

> As soon as . . . the floor was open to discussion, Leake was on his feet. I want to tell you, he was hot under the collar. He presented clinical evidence to the effect that the Kolmer live-virus caused several deaths in children and then point-blank accused Kolmer of being a murderer. All hell broke loose. . . . Jimmy Leake used the strongest language that I ever heard used at a scientific meeting.[70]

Leake had submitted another inquiry to Treasury Department attorneys. He had drafted a statement about Kolmer's vaccine, and he wanted to know if its publication would make him vulnerable to a libel suit.[71] A substantially revised version of Leake's statement would appear in the December 28 issue of *JAMA*.[72] Without naming the vaccine's creators, Leake's published comments made it clear that the two recently introduced immunizing agents were dangerous. The text described cases of post-vaccination polio and discussed the unlikelihood that they were triggered by natural polio. Leake's wording carefully avoided the implication that any specific case of polio among vaccine recipients was caused by immunization. His argument was that the total number of cases could not have been caused by chance or by prior exposure to infantile paralysis. Leake's original draft of the statement addressed Kolmer's vaccine only.[73]

Constructing Unacceptable Risk

The research community had reached a consensus about Kolmer's vaccine, but uncertainty remained about Brodie's preparation. Many scientists continued to question the effectiveness of Brodie's vaccine, although they thought it was probably safe. In early November, Park acknowledged one case of paralytic polio among the recipients of Brodie's preparation in which the timing of paralysis raised questions about the vaccine's involvement. In

Park's view, the case resulted from the vaccine's failure to immunize. Rivers had voiced concerns about Brodie's efforts to improve the vaccine's efficacy by shortening the formaldehyde treatment during production. But after talking with Brodie about the new preparation methods, Rivers judged them to be safe.[74] Nonetheless, in late November, California public health officials received notification of two cases of paralytic polio in Kern County among children who had been vaccinated in October with Brodie's vaccine. The state health department asked Karl Meyer, a Hooper Institute researcher and recipient of PBBC funding, to investigate. Meyer examined medical records on the two cases and concluded that Brodie's vaccine was very probably the source of the infections. He informed Leake of his assessment.[75] Leake then proceeded to include discussion of Brodie's immunizing agent (referred to as "vaccine B") and the California cases in his statement for *JAMA*.

If Meyer and Leake were persuaded that Brodie's vaccine was unsafe, others dissented. Early in 1936, community physicians who had administered Brodie's vaccine in southern California protested the decision to discontinue its use. An editorial in *JAMA* declared that "the case against the formaldehyde vaccine (Brodie) is considered by many to be inconclusive and too hastily drawn."[76] McCoy stated that the cause of paralysis in the two California cases was not amenable to proof.[77] But it was clearly Leake's and McCoy's intention to stop use of both vaccines. The impact of Leake's *JAMA* article would be to curtail demand for the immunizing agents. Leake directed his statement to medical practitioners who might consider using the vaccines. After its publication, the Public Health Service distributed copies to state and municipal public health officials. The article made it clear that the immunizing agents were too dangerous for human use. Nevertheless, Leake had worded the text so that it would not be useful in a vaccine-injury suit or leave Public Health Service scientists vulnerable to legal action for libel.[78]

Meanwhile, the Medical Advisory Committee of the PBBC instructed Park to stop all human use of Brodie's vaccine. The decision was made at a December 13 meeting and McCoy's was the determinative voice. McCoy's primary rationale was not cases of post-vaccination polio but, rather, the "alarming reactions" to foreign tissue in the vaccine. De Kruif recounted McCoy's position on the matter:

> McCoy said that if we went on with our plan to vaccinate a hundred thousand children with this vaccine, in its crude, unpurified state, he would predict a certain number of alarming reactions, some of which might be fatal.

. . . This regardless of the possible immunizing power of the vaccine, alone
would have made it necessary for us to retrace our steps, and seek a more
pure, concentrated vaccine, free of the possibly dangerous monkey nervous
tissue.[79]

Park did not accept the decision gracefully. In the weeks before and after
the December meeting, he lobbied members of the PBBC Advisory Committee for continued support of Brodie's vaccine. He argued that severe constitutional reactions were unavoidable in a small number of cases:

As far as the anaphylactic conditions, I suppose that we would have to expect one in 10,000 to have a severe and possibly fatal result. I went through
this with diphtheria immunization where, as you know, one in about
60,000 died from anaphylactic shock.[80]

He pointed to promising data from field tests—apparently unaware of the
two cases of polio among California recipients—and the lack of other interventions against poliomyelitis:

It is almost certainly true that eighty per cent of the children developed humoral antibodies after two doses of the vaccine and that there have been at
least six cases developing poliomyelitis among the controls [and] only one
case after vaccination. As we have nothing else in view do you not agree
with me that it is worthwhile to go further with the vaccine?[81]

Park complained that Leake's *JAMA* article was unfair in combining cases
from the Kolmer and the Brodie vaccines. Milbank, who concurred, wrote to
McCoy about newspaper coverage of Leake's report:

I judged from what you said at the [Medical Advisory Committee] meeting
that you did not consider the two vaccines in the same category—at least as
regards to the danger attendant upon their use, and it seems unfortunate
that the reports came out in such a way that associated them in this respect
so closely in the public mind.[82]

The reality of deaths attributable to Kolmer's vaccine and the possibility
of additional reactions to Brodie's preparation heightened the research community's awareness of the potential for further devastating outcomes. Public eagerness for an intervention against polio had encouraged the inauguration of clinical testing of polio vaccines. Now the anticipation of public

reaction to fatalities had become a factor in the decision to terminate use of Brodie's vaccine. The two immunizing agents were highly visible to the public. Large numbers of children had received the preparations, and the popular press had covered the vaccines' introduction and diffusion. The publication of Leake's article in *JAMA* would bring outside attention to the vaccine fatalities. Failure to act would likely undermine medical researchers' legitimacy and the public's trust in other immunizing agents. In private correspondence, Karl Meyer alluded to the possibility of a lay inquiry into the vaccine injuries.

Meyer made his remarks in a letter to Joe Smith, head of the health department in Kern County, where Brodie's vaccine had been used during outbreaks of poliomyelitis. Meyer chided Smith for failing to record the lot numbers of the vaccine used in inoculating the two children who later contracted paralytic polio. With information on lot numbers, researchers could have determined whether the sickened children had received vaccine produced with the shortened formaldehyde treatment. Furthermore, vaccine from these lots might have been administered to monkeys to see if it generated paralysis in animals. Meyer told Smith that the vaccine had almost certainly caused the cases of polio. The only acceptable justification for such an outcome would be that it had taken place in the context of a carefully controlled experiment:

> It is most unfortunate that no records of the lots of the vaccine are available. . . . It was my understanding that the mass inoculation as practiced in your county, would be conducted as a carefully planned experiment with detailed records concerning the lots of the vaccines, etc. Valuable information would thus be furnished Drs. Brodie and Park in order to guide them in perfecting the method of immunization. . . . [Use of the vaccines] is only justifiable provided they are conducted as well controlled experiments.[83]

Meyer then invoked the specter of a public investigation of the vaccine-related deaths:

> A lay investigation would promptly stigmatize the inoculations as the cause of the disease and blame the vaccine. . . . I hope you will agree with me that an adverse verdict would place in jeopardy the various recognized vaccination programs against diphtheria, smallpox, etc. aside from being most embarrassing to those who labor in the field of Public Health.[84]

Public scrutiny of vaccine deaths could have damaging consequences not only for public health programs but also for institutions of medical science. Concerns about the prospect of a lay investigation were not unrealistic. The two vaccines had already been the subject of an informal inquiry. In October of 1934, First Lady Eleanor Roosevelt had asked the surgeon general's office to investigate reports that scientists were testing experimental polio vaccines on orphans. She had received letters of protest following the appearance of newspaper articles on the subject. The assistant surgeon general asked Kolmer and Brodie to respond to the allegations and then relayed their responses to the White House.[85]

NIH, constrained by its limited regulatory mandate, could not bring he Kolmer and Brodie vaccines to a halt. When McCoy and Leake moved to end use of the immunizing agents, they were acting not as federal officials but as leaders of the scientific community. They were well positioned to exert such leadership. NIH was a highly respected research laboratory, and McCoy also headed the scientific advisory board of the organization funding Brodie's vaccine. Other powerful figures in the polio-research community supported the actions taken by Leake and McCoy. Scientists had reached a consensus that Kolmer's vaccine was inherently unsafe. Disagreements about Brodie's vaccine remained. But given the deaths from Kolmer's vaccine, serious questions about the safety of Brodie's preparation could not be tolerated.

Scientists' subsequent discussions of the Kolmer and Brodie trials invoked a language of moral violation. I mentioned earlier Rivers's report that, at the St. Louis APHA meetings, Leake had called Kolmer a murderer.[86] De Kruif, in a letter to PBBC officials and supporters, described Park as a scientist "whose age renders him incapable of supervising the work in question" and Brodie as "a man who is not to be trusted."[87] John Paul, just beginning his career as a polio researcher in the early 1930s, emphasized the costs of the vaccine-related deaths of 1934–35 for the next generation of polio researchers:

> The events of 1935 cut more deeply into progress in the immunization of man against poliomyelitis than most people realized at the time. It put an immediate stop to human vaccine trials that was to last for more than fifteen years—so dramatically and traumatically had research programs of a whole generation of investigators on the immunization problem been jolted.[88]

Scientists' discourse depicted the human use of an unsafe clinical intervention as a serious violation against the research community.

The Equivocal Character of Professional Controls

Clinical-research communities make continual assessments about the moral acceptability of human experiments. They base their judgments on the evaluation of empirical evidence bearing on the risks and benefits of the intervention in question. Researchers' judgments are an outgrowth of local knowledge and inseparable from their understandings of the technical content of science. The moral undercurrent in scientists' discourse may be unapparent to outsiders because of the language in which it is couched. Whether a researcher can accurately titrate one minimum paralyzing dose of poliovirus hardly seems like a moral issue to the uninitiated. But questions of this sort may very well be moral-laden to the scientists debating them. Answers to them have bearing on assessments of both the validity of empirical evidence and experimental risks and benefits. Scientists make distinctions between acceptable and unacceptable experiments on this basis.

If, as I have argued, problem groups make moral judgments, why did the polio-research community wait so long before ending the use of Kolmer's vaccine? If investigators thought the preparation was unsafe, why did they fail to act before deaths had occurred? Scientific uncertainty was undoubtedly a contributing factor. Successful vaccine innovation has depended to a large degree on trial and error.[89] There was the possibility that, despite Kolmer's inexperience with poliovirus, he had stumbled upon a solution to the problem of creating a safe and effective polio vaccine. If he had, and others tried to stop the use of his immunizing agent, post hoc judgments would likely have cast Kolmer as farsighted and his critics as lacking vision or motivated by professional jealousy.

Events surrounding termination of the vaccines' use point to the limitations of problem groups as sites for managing investigatory hazards. Research networks are bearers of moral traditions. Their members have specialized scientific expertise requisite for evaluating the likely hazards and benefits of experimental interventions. But there is seldom a level of agreement within investigatory communities that would make collective action easy. Unanimity is difficult to achieve and harder to sustain. This is the reason that clinical moratoria are notoriously unstable. Given the difficulty in achieving consensus about scientific issues, it is not surprising that it is often concern about public reactions to research accidents that triggers the postponement or curtailment of human experiments.

Research networks are informal groups, poorly equipped to impose coercive constraints on their members. Their principal means of social control are granting and withholding esteem and ostracizing those who violate collective norms. When such measures fail to have the intended effect, leaders who wish to take action must do so through their impact on formal organizations or on groups outside the research community. McCoy wielded influence through his position on the advisory board of a vaccine's sponsor. Leake wielded his through his impact on public health workers and medical practitioners—the professionals who administer immunizing agents. Unable to cut off supply of Kolmer's vaccine, he took action that would end demand. But there were costs to Leake's strategy. It would inevitably publicize vaccine deaths and contribute to a heightened perception of the risks of immunizing agents.[90] Implementing moral boundaries could be better handled by the formal organizations that provide support for vaccine trials.

3

Research Sponsors and the Culture of Risk

In the field of vaccine testing, organizational support for human trials was quite common in the United States, even as early as the 1930s. A diverse array of agencies provided resources for the testing of new immunizing agents during the middle third of the twentieth century. These included public health departments, research institutes, private foundations, voluntary associations, pharmaceutical companies, and federal agencies—both civilian and military.[1] By midcentury, sponsors were taking an increasingly active role in regulating the risks entailed in human experiments. Even before World War II, some research sponsors, though by no means all, imposed constraints on the conduct of hazardous vaccine trials.

From the point of view of effecting social control, sponsors have undoubted advantages over scientific problem groups. Even when a colleague network is able to reach agreement about what constitutes undue risk, it may have difficulty controlling the conduct of members. As the 1934–35 polio-vaccine controversy has shown, if informal sanctions fail to deter a scientist considered by peers to be too tolerant of risk, the network alone lacks leverage to enforce its moral judgments. Organizational sponsors do not share this limitation. With control over resources necessary to the conduct of research, sponsors can quickly bring clinical trials to a halt. At the same time, sponsors have varied dramatically in their approaches toward hazards and their inclination to regulate investigatory conduct. In the years between 1935 and 1955, sponsors of vaccine trials undertook support of similar and sometimes concurrent experiments but adopted strikingly different approaches toward the potential for human injury.

In this chapter, I examine how sponsors addressed research hazards and the processes giving rise to their divergent stances. I argue that several organizational dynamics affected a sponsor's oversight policies: decision makers' knowledgeability about the science underlying vaccine development; their experience with investigatory controversy; and incentives for undertaking and avoiding risk created by the organization's distinctive institutional niche. My analysis reveals that the factors influencing research conduct extend well beyond the moral inclinations of individual scientists and the constructions negotiated within professional networks. Organizational dynamics far removed from the research setting have importantly affected whether and how human research proceeds. Clarification of these dynamics sheds light not only on the testing of experimental medical interventions but also the social management of risk-laden technologies more generally.

Divergent Stances toward Research Hazards

I suggest that sponsors' stances toward hazards can be understood as falling into three general patterns: *risk avoidance, risk containment,* and *risk delegation. Risk avoidance* occurs where organizational decision makers consider but then decline to support a hazardous human experiment. *Risk containment* occurs where a sponsor proceeds with support for a clinical trial, but imposes measures for monitoring risks and controlling the possible impact of human injury. *Risk delegation* occurs where a sponsor provides research support without taking measures for overseeing risk or controlling its potential consequences. The organization is, in effect, deferring decisions about risk assumption to the individual researcher. For the purpose of this discussion, I consider sponsors that delegate decisions about experimental hazards to be risk tolerant, and those that take action to avoid or contain hazards to be risk averse.

My account focuses on three groups of vaccine trials conducted during the middle third of the twentieth century. The first group of experiments includes the two polio vaccines that proceeded to human testing in 1934–35. In the second group, also dating from the mid-1930s, researchers conducted human inoculations with live influenza virus. In the third group, dating from the 1950s, investigators initiated human trials of new live-polio vaccines. In each set of experiments, two or more research teams, working contemporaneously but under different auspices, conducted—or considered conducting—an immunization experiment. In each, the preparations being tested were directed against the same disease. Yet in each, sponsors adopted very different approaches to the possibility of human injury. The actual and perceived dangers of the vaccines alone do not account for these differences. Indeed, it was sometimes a sponsor of the least hazardous immunizing agent that took the greatest precautions against risk. Moreover, where multiple agencies supported a single trial, the organizations often diverged in their responses to the potential for human harm (see table 1 for a summary of the vaccine trials discussed here, the trials' sponsors, and these sponsors' stances toward risk).

The Polio-Vaccine Trials of 1934–1935

In chapter 2, I described the short-lived human use of the Park-Brodie and the Kolmer vaccines. The immunizing agent developed by William Park and Maurice Brodie at the New York City Health Department Laboratory was a killed-virus preparation. John Kolmer's preparation, developed at the Institute for Cutaneous Medicine (ICM) in Philadelphia, was a live-virus vaccine. Both research teams began clinical tests in the summer of 1934. Each conducted initial human trials and then released its preparation to physicians and public health agencies for use on an experimental basis. According to the vaccines' creators, thousands of individuals received one of the two immunizing agents. But the vaccines' use came to a halt in the late fall of 1935, following reports that recipients of Kolmer's preparation had contracted paralytic polio. Prominent members of the research community had reached a consensus that Kolmer's vaccine had generated the disease it was designed to prevent, and that Brodie's preparation was triggering troubling allergic reactions.

Patterns of sponsorship for the Park-Brodie vaccine were complex. The scientists prepared their immunizing agent and conducted animal tests at the City of New York Health Department Laboratory, where Park was director. Both Park and Brodie also held appointments at the New York University School of Medicine, and it was this institution that administered external funding for polio-vaccine development. Park secured support from three outside sources: the New York Foundation; the Rockefeller Foundation; and, beginning in 1935, the President's Birthday Ball Commission (PBBC).[2]

Kolmer also had multiple sponsors. He produced his vaccine at the ICM, the entrepreneurial laboratory that he headed. A research fund at the Temple University School of Medicine, where Kolmer held an appointment, provided additional support. After testing his preparation in clinical trials for a number of months, Kolmer negotiated an arrangement for manufacturing

Table 1. Sponsors' Stances toward Risk

Investigator and Sponsor	Organizational Behavior	Approach to Risk
COMPARISON 1: 1934–1935 POLIO VACCINE TRIALS		
Park and Brodie		
NYC Health Department Laboratory	Allows investigators to proceed with clinical use of risky vaccine, apparently leaving decisions to the researchers.	Delegation
New York Foundation	Provides support for vaccine research without oversight or risk-mangaement measures.	Delegation
Rockefeller Foundation's IHD	Provides support for vaccine research after scientific evaluation but with no risk-management measures.	Delegation
PBBC	Advisory panel first approves and then ends support for risky clinical trial.	Containment
Kolmer		
ICM	Allows investigator to proceed with clinical use of very risky vaccine; declines to stop use in the face of injuries.	Delegation
Temple University Neurology Fund	Provides support for vaccine research apparently without oversight or risk-management measures.	Delegation
PBBC	Advisory panel declines to support very risky clinical trial.	Avoidance
Kramer*		
Rockefeller Foundation's IHD	Provides support for vaccine research after scientific evaluation but with no risk-management measures.	Delegation
Flexner*		
Rockefeller Institute	Organizational culture discourages researcher from proceeding with risky clinical trial.	Avoidance
COMPARISON 2: 1935–1937 INFLUENZA-VIRUS TRIALS		
Francis		
Rockefeller Institute	Allows investigator to conduct risky trial after scientific evaluation and with multiple risk-management measures.	Containment
Stokes		
Abington Memorial Hospital Fund	Provides support for vaccine research apparently without oversight or risk-management measures.	Delegation
U.S. Department of Agriculture	Provides support for vaccine research apparently without oversight or risk-management measures.	Delegation
Rockefeller Foundation's IHD	Provides support for vaccine research after scientific evaluation but with no risk-management measures.	Delegation

(continued)

Table 1. (*Continued*)

Investigator and Sponsor	Organizational Behavior	Approach to Risk
COMPARISON 3: 1950S LIVE-POLIO VACCINE TRIALS		
Koprowski		
Lederle Laboratories	Allows researcher to proceed with use of very risky vaccine apparently without risk-management measures.	Delegation
Sabin		
National Foundation	Advisory panels approve clinical use of risky vaccine. Sponsor imposes multiple risk-management measures.	Containment

*Researcher did not proceed to human testing.

the immunizing agent with the William S. Merrill pharmaceutical corporation.[3] Early in 1935, the PBBC had discussed funding for Kolmer's work, but a key member of its scientific board considered the live-polio vaccine too hazardous for human testing.[4]

Historical documents reveal a clear pattern in how sponsors approached research hazards. The PBBC was risk averse in its stance toward both the Park-Brodie and the Kolmer vaccines. All other sponsors of the two immunizing agents delegated decisions about risk assumption to the vaccines' creators. The PBBC engaged in risk containment with Park and Brodie's vaccine, cutting off funding to the researchers when the organization's scientific advisors became alarmed about allergic reactions and several suspicious cases of polio among vaccine recipients. It was this action by the PBBC scientific board that ended human use of the immunizing agent. Neither the New York Foundation nor the Rockefeller Foundation made an effort to affect use of the Park-Brodie preparation.[5] Meanwhile, the PBBC displayed risk avoidance toward Kolmer's vaccine, by declining to fund his research. In this context, the behavior of Kolmer's sponsors, particularly the ICM, is especially striking. The ICM failed to deter Kolmer from continuing human use of his immunizing agent even after members of the research community had confronted him with evidence that the vaccine was causing paralytic polio.[6] Thus, for some time, neither Kolmer nor his sponsors ended use of his vaccine, despite what contemporary scientists considered to be overwhelming evidence that the preparation was dangerous.

Another contrast also merits further comment. As discussed in chapter 2, the researchers who began human polio-vaccine testing in 1934 were not the only ones working with experimental immunizing agents against poliomyelitis. At least two other investigators had the capability of conducting human trials of such agents but chose not to do so: Sidney D. Kramer at Long Island Medical College (LIMC) and Simon Flexner at the Rockefeller Institute. Kramer had moved to LIMC in 1934, where, with the help of a senior member of the medical faculty, he secured funding from the Rockefeller Foundation for polio-vaccine studies. His immunizing agent was composed of poliovirus neutralized with convalescent serum.[7] Flexner had developed and conducted animal tests with numerous experimental polio vaccines during the 1910s. He returned to the problem of polio immunity in the late 1920s and early 1930s, overseeing work on immune sera and testing a newly evolved attenuated strain of polio on monkeys.[8]

Personal moral inclinations undoubtedly played a role in decisions by Kramer and Flexner to refrain from human trials. Both researchers took the high ground on matters of professional conduct. Kramer made a number of statements suggesting that he was personally committed to avoiding risky human experiments.[9] In 1932, the *New York Times* reported that researchers at Harvard were conducting laboratory tests with a new immunizing agent against poliomyelitis. A reporter asked Kramer, then working at Harvard in Lloyd Aycock's laboratory, whether the preparation would undergo human testing. According to the *Times*, Kramer responded, "The Pasteur age is over. There can be no more disastrous wholesale experiments like Pasteur's rabies treatments to children before the serum was wholly proved."[10] Interestingly, Kramer's published remark won him a rebuke from Rockefeller Institute scientists concerned about state legislative efforts of antivivisection activists.[11] Available records are silent on the matter of Kramer's thoughts about inaugurating human tests of the neutralized poliovirus he developed while at LIMC. But the requirements of his sponsor were apparently not a factor. Records of the Rockefeller Foundation contain no indication that it expressed an opinion about the clinical testing of his 1934 anti-polio preparation.[12]

A clearer picture emerges of Flexner's decision making. Flexner had long assumed a position of moral stewardship within the research community, working to promote scientific medicine and protect its institutions from antivivisectionist attacks on animal and human experimentation. In resisting human trials, Kramer and Flexner were conforming to a clinical moratorium that Flexner himself had spearheaded in the early 1910s. Nonetheless, Flexner is unambiguous that, in the decision to refrain from conducting human tests of polio vaccines, institutional considerations were important as well. He made a statement to this effect in a note to Peyton Rous, in March 1935. Rous had asked Flexner to review the paper that Maurice Brodie had submitted to the *Journal of Experimental Medicine*. In his communication to Rous about Brodie's submission, Flexner commented on Park and Brodie's decision to proceed with human testing:

> Park did a good job in removing the fear to try modified poliomyelitis virus as an immunizing agent in children. We could have done this years ago, but I was afraid, since any accident—an intercurrent poliomyelitis case— would have cost the [Rockefeller] Institute too dearly and injured the cause of animal experimentation. Park as a city official was protected, besides which he is far more fearless of human consequences than I am.[13]

Flexner's remarks reveal the multiple influences affecting his decision to continue the moratorium on clinical testing. Fear of human consequences and protection of the research community from antivivisectionist attacks weighed heavily. So too did the well-being of the Rockefeller Institute. Here Flexner was acting in his capacity as scientific director in the interest of sparing the Institute's reputation. In short, as a Rockefeller Institute leader, Flexner adopted risk avoidance as a stance toward the hazards of human experimentation.

The Influenza-Virus Inoculations of 1935 – 1937

During the mid-1930s, two scientists, working independently, injected human subjects with live-influenza preparations. One of the researchers was Joseph Stokes Jr., who was beginning a career in academic medicine at the University of Pennsylvania and Philadelphia Children's Hospital. The other was Thomas Francis Jr., a young investigator on the scientific staff of the Rockefeller Institute. The organizations supporting Stokes's work made no attempt to influence his investigatory procedures and apparently took little notice of the hazards involved in his research. In contrast, as Francis's sponsor, the Rockefeller Institute closely monitored his research and imposed numerous procedures designed to control risks to both his subjects and the Institute itself. Sponsors of the two trials differed dramatically in their approach to investigatory hazards—this despite the fact that the two researchers were using the same immunizing agent.[14]

Francis and Stokes were pursuing different goals in conducting human inoculations with live influenza. Francis was completing a series of studies isolating and identifying a specific virus as a cause of influenza. In earlier experiments, Francis had transferred human influenza to ferrets, replicating the work of the British researchers who had first created an animal model of the disease.[15] Francis's human inoculations were scientifically important because they confirmed that his viral strain, having been cultivated in animals, would generate antibodies against influenza in the human body. Before conducting the clinical trial, Francis passed the virus through ferrets and mice and cultivated it in a tissue-culture media. He expected that these procedures would attenuate the strength of the virus.[16] Francis conducted his first human inoculations in September and October of 1935, injecting fourteen subjects with the viral strain. A second set of inoculations expanded the recipient pool to twenty-three subjects. Francis tested subjects' antibody levels before and after the inoculations. He found that the injected virus in fact stimulated circulating antibodies and that it did so without generating clinical symptoms.[17]

Stokes's purpose was to assess the utility of the viral strain as an immunizing agent. In his initial clinical experiments, Stokes conducted human inoculations with both human and swine flu viruses. He obtained the viral strains from Rockefeller Institute scientists—the human virus from Francis, and the swine flu from Richard Shope at the Institute's New Jersey laboratory. During the fall of 1935, Stokes's team tested the human virus on several members of the hospital staff and on a handful of patients.[18] In February of 1936, they proceeded with a clinical trial at a state custodial institution. There, 110 subjects received human virus, 138 received swine virus, and 550 inmates served as unvaccinated controls. The researchers assessed subjects' antibody levels before and after inoculations and confirmed that both viruses stimulate antibody production. Stokes then proceeded with a study designed to assess whether inoculations would protect recipients from natural exposure to influenza. In the winter of 1936–37, his collaborators administered immunizations of human virus to one third of the inmates at each of five custodial facilities. Seventeen hundred subjects received immunizations while 3,300 remained unvaccinated. Outbreaks of influenza occurred at two of the institutions. Stokes reported that the incidence of severe respiratory illness was lower among vaccinated subjects than among unvaccinated controls.[19]

Patterns of sponsorship for work by the two investigators differed markedly. The Rockefeller Institute was the sole sponsor of Francis's initial influenza-inoculation experiment. In addition to providing salary and routine research support, the Institute allocated $2,100 for Francis's trial from its contingency fund.[20] Stokes cobbled together funding from a number of sources. Hospital charitable donations provided the initial resources. Beginning in July of 1935, Stokes received about $2,300 per year for influenza research from a charitable fund at Abington Memorial Hospital, where he held a courtesy appointment. He used this donation to cover salaries for laboratory assistants.[21] In 1936, Stokes secured $2,500 per year for work on swine flu from the Bureau of Animal Industry of the U.S. Department of Agriculture. This resulted from his involvement in a collaborative project initiated by faculty at the University of Pennsylvania Veterinary School.[22] Stokes also obtained a grant of $12,000 from the Rockefeller Foundation for the clinical testing of the influenza virus.[23]

Francis's and Stokes's sponsors had strikingly different stances toward the dangers of inoculating human subjects with an experimental immunizing agent. The Rockefeller Institute actively engaged in risk containment. Members of its Board of Scientific Directors had extensive discussions about the advisability of conducting an experiment like Francis's under the Institute's auspices. They also sought the opinion of Rufus Cole, head of the Institute's hospital, where subjects were to be housed in isolation during the trial. The experiment was problematic in part because, in response to antivivisectionist protest earlier in the century, the Rockefeller Institute Hospital had made it an explicit policy to refrain from conducting experiments on patients. Homer Swift, an investigator at the hospital and an advocate for Francis's experiment among the Institute's leadership, acknowledged "the peculiar position of the Rockefeller Institute in such a procedure."[24] But he insisted that the scientific gain from the experiment justified the hazards. Swift wrote to Flexner saying that, concerns about human experimentation at the Institute notwithstanding, "the final test must be carried out on men and . . . if we safeguard ourselves by using physicians or medical students the results should be worth the risks."[25] Senior researchers at the Institute permitted Francis's trial to proceed because they agreed with Swift about its scientific significance.

While allowing Francis to conduct human inoculations, the Institute's leaders closely oversaw his experiment and imposed a number of procedural requirements. They made sure that before the human trial began, Francis had conducted all appropriate animal experiments. They insisted— as suggested in Swift's statement to Flexner—that Francis's subjects be either physicians or medical students. They had Francis use an elaborate consent form, written by lawyers, that released the Institute from liability for injury to subjects.[26] They required subjects to be held in quarantine during the experiment—an isolation ward at the Rockefeller Institute Hospital was opened for this purpose. They delayed Francis's trial until the hospital director, Rufus Cole, was back from vacation.[27] Finally, they placed restrictions on how Francis was to perform the inoculations. Swift instructed Francis to inject the virus, a procedure expected to stimulate antibodies without symptoms, rather than expose subjects' nasal mucosa, viewed as more likely to generate clinical infection.[28]

In contrast, organizations supporting Stokes's research had little to say about the risks of human testing, and they imposed no procedural requirements.[29] Instead, they left all decisions about risk assumption to Stokes and his research team. In selecting human subjects, Stokes followed a course common among early- and mid-twentieth-century vaccine researchers, conducting clinical trials with the inmates of custodial institutions. Stokes located his first human experiment (begun in February 1936) at the New Jersey State Colony in New Lisbon, a facility housing "eight hundred feeble-minded males."[30] Trials during the winter of 1936–37 took place at four additional custodial facilities in New Jersey, including a state correctional facility for boys, a home for epileptics, and two other institutions for the mentally disabled.[31]

I found no discussion of Stokes's choice of subjects in either the Rockefeller Foundation files on his project or in his correspondence with other backers. Nor did these sponsors raise the issue of subjects' consent for participation in research. As will be discussed further in chapter 4, during the early decades of the twentieth century, it was often the managers of custodial institutions providing access to subjects—not an investigator's sponsors—who required consent and raised questions about risks.[32] What the Rockefeller Foundation's records do show is that the organization viewed Stokes's access to large numbers of institutionalized subjects as an opportunity for evaluating the effectiveness of available influenza strains in generating immunity. The Foundation's International Health Division (IHD) was willing to provide Stokes with support given that opening. Nevertheless, it was quick to terminate Stokes's funding—it did so in June of 1938—when the accumulated data indicated that the viruses were inadequate for widespread application. The Rockefeller Foundation may have delegated decisions about experiments with institutionalized subjects—an isolated population—to the individual scientist, but it was careful to forestall broader distribution of a vaccine it viewed as inappropriate for general use.[33]

The Testing of Live-Polio Vaccines in the 1950s

In a third set of vaccine trials, two investigators proceeded with the human testing of newly developed live-polio vaccines. Hilary Koprowski began a series of clinical experiments with attenuated polio strains early in 1950. His sponsor and employer—Lederle Laboratories, the pharmaceutical division of American Cyanamid Company—carried all of Koprowski's research expenses. Five years later, Albert Sabin inaugurated human testing of his own polio strains. Sabin held appointments at the University of Cincinnati

Medical School and the Cincinnati Children's Hospital. His sole source of funding was the National Foundation for Infantile Paralysis. As I describe shortly, the organizations supporting development and testing of the two vaccines diverged sharply in their stances toward investigatory hazards.

In the fifteen years that followed the Kolmer and Park-Brodie trials, laboratory research on poliomyelitis created the basis for a new generation of polio vaccines. Scientists identified three antigenetically distinct types of polio and greatly expanded knowledge of variation among strains. They discovered that infected individuals excrete polio in their stools and that the virus is passed from person to person via fecal-oral contamination. They created methods for infecting rodents with polio and for growing the virus in non-neurologic tissue cultures. By the late 1940s, a good number of researchers were working on the development of experimental polio vaccines. Some, like Jonas Salk, focused their efforts on killed-virus preparations. Others felt that only an attenuated live virus would generate lasting immunity.[34] The availability of rodent models and tissue cultures provided a range of techniques for cultivating attenuated viral strains that might be suitable immunizing agents. The problem was to develop attenuated strains that would generate immunity without symptoms and that would also remain benign to the contacts of vaccine recipients.

Koprowski announced the results of his first human trial of live polio strains at a roundtable conference held by the National Foundation in March 1951.[35] Members of the research community were astonished to learn that he had proceeded with a clinical experiment. Since the unsuccessful trials of 1934–35, no scientist had admitted to inoculating humans with any polio vaccine, let alone a live-virus preparation.[36] Jonas Salk did not begin the human testing of his killed-virus vaccine until July of 1952. Contemporary researchers were, at best, doubtful of the appropriateness of Koprowski's human experiment. By Koprowski's own account, many considered the inoculations "not only perilous for the subjects of the trial but also as sinful on the part of the investigators."[37] In the end, the research community judged Koprowski's early strains to be too hazardous for general distribution. In 1956, Koprowski release his Type I and Type II stains to investigators in Belfast, who conducted their own human trials with the viruses. These researchers found that Koprowski's strains, when excreted by vaccine recipients, reverted toward increased virulence. The excreted viruses caused paralysis in some monkeys. Koprowski's early preparations might have been safe for the vaccines' recipients, but the Belfast studies suggested that individuals in close proximity to these recipients were at risk for contracting paralytic polio.[38]

Koprowski's initial human clinical trial took place at Letchworth Village, a facility for disabled children run by the New York State Department of Mental Hygiene. Between February 1950 and January 1951, his team fed an attenuated polio strain to twenty inmates with no prior immunity to the virus. The strain tested at Letchworth was a Type II poliovirus attenuated by passage through rodents—the TN strain developed by Koprowski's assistant, Thomas Norton. The researchers reported that the vaccine stimulated antibodies—as well as virus in subjects' stool—without generating clinical symptoms.[39] The following year, Koprowski inoculated sixty additional children with the TN strain, this time at Sonoma State Hospital in California. In 1954–55, he tested strains of both Type II and Type I polio at several custodial facilities, including Sonoma State (providing seventy subjects) and the State Colony at Woodbine in New Jersey (providing twenty-four subjects). In 1955–56, he added a Type III strain, which he tested at Clinton Farms, a state facility for delinquent girls in New Jersey.[40]

By that time, Sabin had begun human trials of his own strains of attenuated live polioviruses. His initial research site was the Chillicothe Federal Reformatory, a facility in Ohio run by the Federal Bureau of Prisons of the U.S. Department of Justice. In January of 1955, Sabin inoculated thirty prisoners—all twenty-one years of age or older—with Types I, II, and III polio strains. Between April 1955 and April 1956, he tested strains of polioviruses on ninety additional adult inmates at Chillicothe. Like Koprowski and his collaborators, Sabin found that subjects developed antibodies and briefly became polio carriers (excreting live virus), while displaying no clinical symptoms of poliomyelitis.[41]

Differences in the sponsors' stances toward the risk of live-polio vaccines were dramatic. Lederle Laboratories engaged in risk delegation, permitting Koprowski broad discretion in his investigatory conduct. Writing in the 1960s about his initial trial of live polio at Letchworth, Koprowski states that apart from his two collaborators, one of whom was medical director at Letchworth, "no one else knew of the study during the period between February 27, 1950, when the first child was fed the virus and late January, 1951, when observation of the first series of 20 subjects was nearing completion."[42] This statement could not have been literally true, since personnel at Letchworth other than the medical director would have known that a clinical trial was in progress. But Koprowski's assertion does suggest that other scientists at Lederle Laboratories were unaware of the experiment until it was over. Lederle permitted Koprowski sufficiently wide latitude that he was able to conduct human tests with live poliovirus years before other postwar researchers, and apparently also without systematic review by senior scientists within its research division. The company did so in the absence of a professional consensus that the viral stains were likely to be safe for human application. Koprowski's publications indicate that he obtained consent to vaccinate children before proceeding with human testing. But it is unclear whether this was a requirement of Lederle Laboratories.[43]

In contrast, the National Foundation sought to contain the dangers of vaccine experiments and insisted that Sabin observe a variety of risk-management procedures. The Foundation used a system of scientific advisory panels to monitor and control the hazards its researchers assumed, requiring that such a panel sign off on human trials before the experiments began. Sabin's proposed human trial underwent formal review by the National Foundation's Vaccine Advisory Committee.[44] Sabin's work also received informal scrutiny from members of the organization's Subcommittee on Live Virus Immunization.[45] Obtaining approvals took the better part of nine months. Sabin requested clearance in March of 1954 and did not receive it until November of that year. In the process, the Foundation's director of research, Henry Kumm, had Sabin respond to detailed questions about his prior animal experiments. This included information on the monkeys Sabin had inoculated—both intracerebrally and intraspinally—with each of his viral strains, as well as the animal tests performed on viruses excreted by inoculated monkeys. Kumm had Sabin specify, in writing, the number of animals undergoing each intervention and the outcome of each procedure.[46] When the Vaccine Advisory Committee granted Sabin approval, its head, Rockefeller Institute scientist Thomas Rivers, stipulated that Sabin could proceed only with the specific cultures the committee had cleared. Sabin would have to seek approval again if he wanted to conduct human tests with new polio strains.[47] Meanwhile, the Foundation's leadership instructed Sabin—and other researchers conducting human trials—to purchase liability insurance.[48] And the Foundation's legal department gave Sabin explicit directions about the wording of consent documents to be used at Chillicothe.[49] In short, the National Foundation was substantially more risk averse than was Lederle Laboratories, this despite the view of contemporary researchers that Sabin's preparations were the safer of the two sets of immunizing agents.

Risk Management as Organizational Policy

Comparison of vaccine trials provides compelling evidence that organizational sponsors diverged markedly in their attention to and precautions against experimental hazards. Most sponsors were risk tolerant, delegating decisions about risk assumption—and other aspects of the moral conduct of research—to the individual investigator. Several were risk averse, declining to sponsor hazardous trials or imposing measures to monitor and contain the impact of risk. Differences in actual or perceived levels of risk, alone, do not account for divergences in sponsors' behavior. In two of the three comparison groups examined in this chapter—those involving immunizing agents against poliomyelitis—it was a sponsor of the vaccine viewed by contemporary researchers as the less hazardous that took greatest precautions. Furthermore, even sponsors backing the same experiment often responded differently to investigatory risk.

Scientists can and do refrain from proceeding with human trials without directives from organizations. Personal conscience was undoubtedly a factor for both Kramer and Flexner when each held back from human trials of polio vaccines. At the same time, archival records show that some sponsors issued explicit instructions to researchers about the conduct of risky experiments. They instituted procedures for handling such experiments and made these procedures official policy. Moreover, where an organization was in a position to support more than one vaccine experiment, there were continuities in its stance across clinical trials. Among the "repeat sponsors," the Rockefeller Foundation's IHD was consistently risk tolerant. In contrast, both the Rockefeller Institute and the PBBC, reconstituted in the late 1930s as the National Foundation, were consistently risk averse.

Accounting for Differences

Organizations' stances toward research hazards were highly consequential for the conduct of vaccine trials. Sponsors affected whether or not a new immunizing agent proceeded to human testing. They determined whether, in light of new concerns about safety, use of a vaccine continued or stopped. They shaped decisions about the selection of subjects and the manner in which experimental immunizations were conducted. If the perceived risk alone does not explain differences in sponsors' approaches to experimental hazards, what does account for this variation? I suggest that three factors merit close scrutiny: decision makers' scientific expertise and their knowledge of investigatory hazards; sponsors' distinctive incentives and disincentives for pursuing risky experiments; and the organization's experience with investigatory controversy. The first of these factors concerns processes internal to organizations. The second two involve organizations' relations with outside constituencies.

Scientific Expertise

The organizations that provided support for human testing of vaccines varied markedly in the extent to which decision makers were familiar with immunization hazards. Sponsors ranged from professional organizations with scientist-managers who had substantial experience with vaccine testing to lay-managed associations without in-house scientific expertise and little or no experience with immunization experiments. Several patterns emerge from my comparison groups regarding knowledgeability and responses to risk (see table 2 for a schematic presentation of these patterns). Not surprisingly, all organizations whose decision makers lacked scientific expertise delegated the management of risk to the researchers it supported. Sponsors in this category include the New York Foundation, the Abington Memorial Hospital Fund, and perhaps also the Temple University Neurology Fund and the animal division of the U.S. Department of Agriculture.[50] The New York Foundation dispensed charitable funds for projects aimed at improvements in education, crime prevention, medical care, and public health. It supported several activities undertaken by New York City's health department, including the creation of a serum laboratory and work on a polio vaccine. The Foundation's trustees, a group composed largely of prominent businessmen, had no expertise in the science underlying immunization research and deferred decisions about technical matters to professionals who directed the projects.[51]

In contrast, sponsors with knowledgeable decision makers varied in their approach toward the risks of human experiments. The two organizations that were consistently risk averse, the Rockefeller Institute and the

Table 2. Sponsors' Knowledgeability and Orientation toward Risk

ORIENTATION TOWARD RISK	ARE DECISION MAKERS KNOWLEDGEABLE?	
	No	Yes
Averse		Rockefeller Institute
		PBBC/National Foundation
Tolerant	New York Foundation	ICM
	Abington Memorial Hospital Fund	NYC Health Department
	Temple University Neurology Fund*	Laboratory
	U.S. Department of Agriculture*	Rockefeller Foundation's IHD
		Lederle Laboratories

*Classification is tentative owing to scarcity of data on decision makers.

PBBC/National Foundation, had ready access to specialized scientific expertise. At the Rockefeller Institute, the Board of Scientific Directors was responsible for decisions about whether and how to proceed with Francis's 1935 influenza-virus trial. The board included both in-house researchers and investigators from other prestigious medical institutions.[52] At the PBBC, lay administrators created a scientific advisory panel to provide oversight and make judgments about funding research protocols. It was this panel that first supported and then terminated human trials of the Park-Brodie vaccine. By the late 1940s, the PBBC—by then renamed the National Foundation—had a scientist serving as full-time research director and several standing committees of polio experts. Advisory panels made many of the decisions about which projects would receive funding. As emphasized earlier, National Foundation policy also required that all investigators working under its aegis obtain formal approval from its one of its scientific committees before proceeding with the human testing of a polio vaccine.

At the same time, four other sponsors with in-house scientific expertise delegated judgments about risk assumption to the individual researcher: the ICM, the New York City Health Department Laboratory, the Rockefeller Foundation's IHD, and Lederle Laboratories. In the case of the first two of these sponsors, the scientist developing the vaccine was also head of the laboratory—explaining, in part, the organizations' confidence in the immunizing agent. The behavior of the other two sponsors, the IHD and Lederle Laboratories, is more perplexing. Why would organizations with ready access to technical knowledge choose to defer decisions about investigatory hazards?

The IHD funded numerous vaccine trials between the mid-1930s and mid-1950s. The organization routinely conducted systematic scientific review of projects under consideration for sponsorship. Division directors were themselves competent medical investigators and division staff regularly obtained opinions about its grantees' work from scientists at the neighboring Rockefeller Institute.[53] Yet unlike the Rockefeller Institute, the IHD imposed no constraints on the conduct of human experiments. As mentioned earlier, the IHD curtailed funding for Stokes when it concluded that the vaccine he was testing was unsuitable for general use. The division assessed the potential public health value of an immunizing agent when making decisions about initiating and terminating external support. But it left to researchers judgments about whether and when to proceed with human testing and how to handle research subjects. The IHD's stance toward investigatory hazards reflected a more general philanthropic policy at the Rockefeller Foundation. Simply put, this policy was that, "once grants are made to responsible groups or institutions, no degree of control over the operation of the grants should be exercised by the foundation."[54] The IHD's reluctance to interfere with ongoing research was a feature of the Rockefeller Foundation's distinctive organizational culture.

Lederle Laboratories, sponsor of Koprowski's polio-vaccine trial, also could call upon substantial in-house scientific expertise but apparently delegated decisions about clinical trials to individual researchers. The company recruited investigators from universities and elite research institutions and prided itself in having a professional research-and-development facility that afforded scientists many of the freedoms available in academic settings.[55] At the time Koprowski conducted his first polio-vaccine trial, he was associate director of Lederle's section on virus research. The section director was Herald Cox, a vaccine investigator who, earlier in his career, had worked on poliomyelitis with Simon Flexner at the Rockefeller Institute. Cox was certainly familiar with the hazards posed by human testing of live polio strains. As noted earlier, Cox and other managers at Lederle were apparently unaware that Koprowski was proceeding with the first human trial of his polio vaccines until the experiment was completed. The author of one account of midcentury polio-vaccine research remarks that "Koprowski acted more or less independently" at Lederle Laboratories. "It was taken for granted that Koprowski was a law unto himself."[56] This episode is a reminder that informal processes can leave even technically expert managers uninformed about hazards being undertaken under the organization's aegis. Where scientists are situated in semiautonomous enclaves within a larger corporate structure, managers, even other scientists, may be unaware of the risks researchers are assuming.[57]

Among the vaccine sponsors examined in this chapter, access to expert knowledge was a necessary but not sufficient condition for the adoption of a risk-averse policy toward research. Decision makers' familiarity with vaccine science explains some but not all of the variation in sponsors' approaches toward the dangers of human experiments. What it does not account for is differences in risk tolerance among the sponsors that had ready access to scientific experts. Thus far, I have suggested that information processes and organizational culture help to account for differences in the behavior of scientifically knowledgeable sponsors. A fuller explanation requires looking outside the organizations to the social context in which sponsors operated.

Incentives and Disincentives

Sociological literature emphasizes the importance of the broader environment in shaping organizational behavior. While scholars differ in how they conceive of the environment, the notion often includes three components: the material and technical resources necessary for the organization to operate; the normative, regulatory, and cultural context; and the network of other organizations that engage in similar activities.[58] Recent theorists argue that organizations within the same institutional sector develop shared notions of appropriate procedures and practices as they interact with each other and respond to social and economic pressures. In this view, interconnected organizations come to share a common environment that they, in part, constitute, and that affects the behavior of constituent organizations.[59] Early- and mid-twentieth-century research sponsors did not entirely conform to this picture of common norms and practices and a shared environment. It is true that these sponsors did function in the same regulatory context—the body of legal rulings bearing on liability for research injuries. They also shared and were connected by networks of scientists who conducted medical experiments. But the organizations that supported early clinical research competed in different markets for prestige and resources. Sponsors operated within several distinct institutional niches, each generating divergent incentives and disincentives for pursing risky human experiments.

I argue that three different incentives provided the central motivation for sponsors knowledgeable about investigatory hazards to proceed with human experiments: recognition for contributions to medical science (in the case of the Rockefeller Institute); recognition for breakthroughs in disease eradication (in the case of the IHD, the PBBC/National Foundation, and the New York City Health Department Laboratory); and rewards from the commercial development of new immunizing agents (in the case of the ICR and Lederle Laboratories). All sponsors sought to avoid human injury and damage to their reputation associated with investigatory controversy. But their unique relations with outside constituencies meant that the possibility of an accident carried different meaning and weight. Examining these distinctive incentives and disincentives helps to explain patterns of risk assumption among sponsors with access to scientific expertise.

The two consistently risk-averse organizations—the Rockefeller Institute and the PBBC/National Foundation—had strong reasons both for avoiding human injury and for proceeding with at least some hazardous experiments. The Rockefeller Institute had deep-seated trepidations about the consequences to the Institute of any illness that might arise among research subjects. Yet it was willing to proceed with Francis's influenza trial because its managers viewed that experiment has having particular scientific importance. The PBBC was also extremely sensitive regarding its public image—

an image linked to the person of an American president. With no permanent endowment, the organization relied entirely on charitable donations
for operating expenses. The PBBC's ability to attract donations and volunteer workers rested on the sustained perception that it was alleviating human suffering.[60] At the same time, securing a vaccine against polio was a
central reason for the organization's existence. Undertaking human experiments with inherently risky viral strains was necessary to achieve this goal.
By mobilizing expert advice, the PBBC's leadership sought to pursue the organization's mission while taking responsible measures to protect both the
potential recipients of experimental vaccines and its own legitimacy. The
PBBC is unusual for being a lay-managed organization that established a
scientific panel to monitor investigatory hazards. Its high degree of dependence on outside resources generated the motivation for doing so. Both the
Rockefeller Institute and the PBBC responded to strong pushes and pulls by
devoting substantial effort to measures for containing risk.

Two other research sponsors with in-house scientific expertise—the
ICM and Lederle Laboratories—are noteworthy for their willingness to be
risk tolerant toward the testing of live polio strains that the scientific community judged to be particularly hazardous. The ICM permitted Kolmer to
make his vaccine available after other researchers had confronted him with
evidence that the preparation was unsafe. Kolmer headed the ICM at the
time, and he was undoubtedly determinative in the organization's position
this matter. But the ICM's market niche may have contributed as well. Originally called the Dermatological Research Laboratory, the ICM had a long
history of "scientific commercialism."[61] As mentioned in chapter 2, its
founders had profited handsomely from the manufacture and sale of Salvarsan during World War I. They sold their manufacturing facility to Abbott
Laboratories and used their windfall of half a million dollars to endow a not-
for-profit research institute.[62] While supporting the investigatory activities
of Kolmer and other founders, the ICM remained entrepreneurial in character. In the mid-1930s, it functioned as a working laboratory—performing
tests for local physicians—as much as a research facility.[63] Kolmer's early
move to join forces with a drug company for production of his polio vaccine
suggests that commercial development was among his central goals.

Events surrounding Kolmer's polio vaccine irrevocably damaged his
standing within the elite circles of American medical science. But these circles were not his principal point of reference. This may well be one of the
reasons why polio researchers' efforts to convince Kolmer to terminate use
of his vaccine were ineffective. Kolmer and the ICM were players in the local
medical community in Philadelphia and did not rely on the national market

for scientific prestige. The failure of Kolmer's polio vaccine apparently impeded neither his medical career in Philadelphia nor the ICM's viability.[64] In 1949, Kolmer donated the ICM's remaining endowment to the Temple University Medical School—a non-elite institution—at which time he received an appointment as head of Temple's Department of Public Health and Preventive Medicine.[65]

For Lederle Laboratories, the prospect for a saleable polio vaccine was clearly a primary incentive for proceeding with risky human experiments. One commentator reports that, during the 1950s, Lederle Laboratories invested $13 million to the development of live-polio vaccines. Profits from successfully developed pharmaceuticals made such expenditures possible. The company's proceeds from sales of the antibiotic Aureomycin reached $61 million for the year 1952 alone.[66] Nonetheless, corporate managers were undertaking a huge financial gamble when investing millions of dollars in the development of polio vaccines that might prove to be commercially unviable. In the context of this financial risk, hazards involved in initial human testing may not have been at the forefront of their concerns. In 1950, research accidents resulting in product liability suits were rare. The first highly visible product liability case involving a vaccine occurred in 1955. The pharmaceutical company, Cutter Laboratories, was sued after distributing batches of the Salk vaccine containing incompletely inactivated poliomyelitis. The Cutter incident did not involve human experimentation. The NIH's biological control laboratory had already approved Salk's immunizing agent, and the vaccine was in general distribution. In part for this reason, the Cutter injuries were numerous: 260 cases of polio and 11 deaths. The episode had the effect of generating greater caution among firms, not about issues related to clinical testing, but rather about the liabilities involved in producing vaccines for mass distribution.[67] For a company heavily invested in polio-vaccine development, as was Lederle, the possibility of an accident during initial, small-scale human trials may have seemed an unfortunate but unavoidable risk on the route to a socially desirable and potentially remunerative medical product. In short, perceptions of their relations with the regulatory and resource environments may have rendered some commercial enterprises more willing than other types of research sponsors to pursue hazardous vaccine experiments.[68]

Experience and Learning

A sponsor's environment and market niche not only generated immediate incentives and disincentives for pursuing hazardous experiments, they affected patterns of risk assumption in another way as well. Through inter-action with outside constituencies, managers developed expectations about whether the organization would be held accountable for researchers' inves-tigatory conduct and whether an accident would have consequences damag-ing for the organization. When sociologists who study responses to techno-logical hazards address organizational learning, they refer to responses to accidents and injuries. Scholars note that organizations learn from such episodes and often make changes once problems are apparent. But these au-thors also emphasize that, in many arenas of technology, accidents are rare and organizations have limited opportunity to accumulate knowledge about their likelihood or character.[69] In the case of the organizations that spon-sored vaccine trials, learning took place not only in response to injuries, but also in response to bad publicity generated by regulatory activists. Encoun-ters with social movements and the popular press were particularly forma-tive. Experience with research controversy was the basis for organizational learning that shaped the sponsors' long-term stance toward risk.

Perhaps nowhere is the impact of organizational learning more evident than with the Rockefeller Institute, an organization that during the 1930s was consistently risk averse. As previously noted, the Institute had been the repeated target of antivivisection protests. On a number of occasions, anti-vivisectionists accused an Institute scientist of abusing research subjects and secured coverage of these allegations in the popular press. The organi-zation's managers found these incidents to be highly damaging and took a variety of measures to prevent their recurrence.[70] Adopting a risk-averse stance toward the hazards of human experiments was one such measure. Institute leaders learned to expect that a research accident would trigger publicity harmful to the organization. As a result, they avoided risky human experiments except on infrequent occasions when they judged the scientific merit of a clinical trial to outweigh the dangers. On these occasions, they en-gaged in risk containment.

The Rockefeller Institute's attitude toward the uncertainties of research contrasts sharply with that of the Rockefeller Foundation, where, as noted earlier, the IHD routinely delegated decisions about risk assumption. The IHD's markedly different experience with outside audiences made its risk-tolerant stance possible. Antivivisectionists targeted the Institute, whose mission was the advancement of medical science, but not the IHD, whose mission was the prevention and treatment of disease. The IHD's encoun-ters with outside constituencies, including the press, gave it no cause to modify its hands-off policy toward investigatory conduct.

Finally, experience with investigatory controversy helps to explain the extensive measures taken by the PBBC/National Foundation during the 1950s to contain the risks of polio-vaccine testing. In the aftermath of the Park-Brodie trials, the organization tightened its position on investigatory hazards. Leaders renamed the organization, removing allusion to the U.S. president from its title. They replaced Paul de Kruif, who had overseen the PBBC's original scientific board, and revamped the organization's advisory panels. Meanwhile, they retained their memory of the Park-Brodie "fiasco." In 1954, when preparing to embark on the field trial of Salk's polio vaccine, the Foundation's head instructed staff to write a report on "the bad vaccine of 1935."[71] The outcome of the Park-Brodie vaccine trial was a formative experience that helped to shape the organization's vigilance in controlling hazards in later polio-vaccine trials. Institutional memory of the failed Park-Brodie vaccine was still alive almost twenty years after use of the immunizing agent had ended.

Organizations and Technological Hazards

That organizations have made determinative judgments about the conduct of medical experiments is consistent with a growing body of scholarship on the management of technological hazards. Sociologists who study risk emphasize that it is often an organization that makes consequential decisions about the uses of modern technology. Organizations distribute a broad array of products apart from drugs and vaccines that, while socially desirable, are also potentially hazardous. Organizations and the experts they employ make judgments about the application of technology in fields as wide ranging as civil engineering, energy production, aviation, and manufacturing. It is within institutional contexts that risks of modern technologies are identified, conceptualized, measured, managed. Social scientists have endeavored to clarify the processes that shape organizations' management of hazards. This scholarship shows that organizations employ professional experts and construct risk analyses that transform uncertainties about hazards into calculable dangers and benefits. It reveals that organizations endeavor to shape pubic constructions of risk and to contain repercussions of technology-induced injuries.[72]

The bulk of existing literature focuses on commonalities across organizations in the management of hazards. Few scholars have compared organizations taking divergent stances toward risk in an effort to identify processes that account for differences.[73] Sponsors of early- and mid-twentieth-century vaccine experiments—organizations that operated, to a large degree, in different institutional environments—have offered a unique opportunity in this regard. Systematic comparisons of vaccine sponsors show that some organizations had better access to scientific expertise than others, but that this alone did not account for all of the variation in sponsors' policies toward risk. Incentives and disincentives created by the organization's distinctive market niche were of central importance in shaping its tolerance for hazards. Sponsors highly dependent upon prestige-sensitive resources were more likely than others to be risk averse. Moreover, some organizations learned to be risk averse, developing institutional memories, not only in response to technology-induced accidents, but also from their experiences with public controversy.

In examining sponsors' market niches, I distinguished organizations seeking recognition for contributions to medical science or public health from those with commercial interests in the development of saleable medical products. My account suggests that financial investments affect an organization's weighting of experimental risks and benefits. At least among the sponsors examined here, the organizations with commercial interests in the development of a new immunizing agent were more willing than other sponsors to proceed with the human testing of vaccines that the research community felt were very hazardous.

4

Formalizing Responses to Research Hazards

Between the mid-1930s and mid-1950s, a discernable shift took place in the organizational management of investigatory hazards. Of the three approaches to research risks adopted by organizational sponsors—containment, avoidance, and delegation—containment emerged as the dominant policy. Other approaches to risk did not disappear. There were still sponsors that delegated decisions to individual researchers or declined to support hazardous trials. But at midcentury, growing numbers of American scientists were observing measures for controlling risk imposed by the organizations supporting their research. Furthermore, risk-containment strategies were becoming more formalized and more similar across organizations. Years before the federal policies that created institutional review boards, a handful of particularly influential organizations and agencies were building the rudiments of a system for handling the risks of human experiments.

The emerging system had two central components, one procedural and the other linguistic and symbolic. On the one hand, sponsors imposed measures affecting the conduct of clinical experiments. These included written consent statements, insurance that would compensate injured subjects, and review of research protocols by panels of scientific advisors. On the other hand, sponsors generated rhetoric and imagery in an effort to shape social constructions of experimental hazards. Larger organizations created public relations departments that formulated depictions of human experiments presented to the press, and through it, the public.

In this chapter, I examine the origins and character of sponsors' risk-containment strategies, exploring how sponsors came to pursue particular approaches to managing risk and why their procedures become increasingly homogenous and formalized. My analysis emphasizes organizational processes. I argue that two such processes fostered the adoption of procedures for handling risk: the rationalization typical of large-scale organizations and the tendency for organizations to import policies and procedures from the environment in an effort to win legitimacy with outside audiences. The advent of federal support for medical research beginning in World War II contributed importantly as well. Government agencies administering wartime funds for clinical experiments were at the forefront of regularizing procedures for managing risk. In developing these arguments, I expand my empirical scope beyond vaccine testing and examine a broader range of clinical research.

My account highlights an apparent contradiction in the oversight of mid-twentieth-century research: at the very time that influential sponsors were adopting measures for monitoring and controlling risk, some were also supporting experiments that were both extremely dangerous and without benefit for subjects. These included studies, conducted under federal auspices, where researchers deliberately infected human subjects with serious infectious diseases. How could a system for containing risk have allowed nontherapeutic interventions expected to cause significant harm to research subjects? Part of the answer lies in the cultural ethos that prevailed in America during World War II and the immediate postwar years. Part lies in the multiple ends that institutionalized risk-containment served. A sponsor's purpose in managing research hazards was not only to protect human subjects. It was also to buffer the organization itself from damage as decision makers pursued research they believed would benefit society at large. In the case of some sponsors, consent procedures were largely ceremonial, acknowledging public sentiment regarding the need for participation in clinical experiments to be voluntary, but with little attention to the substance of this injunction.

Wartime and Postwar Research Sponsors

With America's entrance into World War II, the U.S. government became a major sponsor of medical research. Both the levels of funding it provided and the mobilization of scientific personnel it triggered were unprecedented. Two defense-related agencies distributed the bulk of federal funds for medical experimentation during the 1940s: the Committee on Medical

Research (CMR) and the Army Epidemiology Board (AEB). These agencies inaugurated a pattern of growing federal support for university-based medical science, with funding dispensed during this period through contracts with academic institutions.

The CMR was a division of the Office of Scientific Research and Development (OSRD), administered within the Executive Office of the President. Franklin Roosevelt created the OSRD—extant between 1941 and 1946—to direct and support civilian scientific contributions to the war effort. The CMR was constituted as a seven-member board of civilian and military medical researchers and administrators. When making policy recommendations, it regularly consulted committees within the medical division of the National Research Council—part of the National Academy of Sciences. The CMR approved funding for projects on a wide range of problems, including research on antibiotic and antipest agents and studies of treatments for wounds, burns, and shock.[1]

The AEB was administered through the Office of the Army Surgeon General. Its purpose was to mobilize civilian scientific assistance in controlling epidemic diseases affecting the military. The AEB organized its work through commissions, each with a roster of scientists and each focused on a category of diseases. A seven-member board of university researchers oversaw the commissions. The War Department dispensed research funds through contracts with the home institutions of commission directors. Reconstituted in 1949 as the Armed Forces Epidemiology Board (AFEB), the agency continued funding for civilian medical scientists in the postwar years.[2] Between 1943 and 1946, the AEB committed $1.7 million in contracts with university researchers. During its tenure, the CMR dispersed $25 million in support for some six hundred research projects.[3] In the words of a contemporary observer, "planned and coordinated medical research had never been essayed on such a scale."[4] Historian David Rothman writes that this influx of federal support transformed medical research in America from a "cottage industry" into a "national program."[5]

At war's end, the government disbanded the OSRD and assigned to the National Institutes of Health (NIH) both remaining CMR grants and the task of dispensing future funding for university-based medical research. In 1947, NIH's research budget was about $8 million, of which half supported the work of in-house scientists. By 1957, the annual budget for its external grants alone was $100 million. In the meantime, after the war, NIH created a research grants division, established a system of study sections (specialized advisory committees) for review of grant applications, and added new institutes—focused on categories of disease—to its organizational structure. It also opened a hospital to serve as a center for in-house clinical research.[6]

Growth in the scale of sponsorship for medical research was not limited to federal agencies. In the immediate postwar years, some private research patrons were emerging as large operations. Perhaps nowhere was this trend more evident than at the National Foundation for Infantile Paralysis. Between 1938 and 1962, the Foundation devoted $69 million to research on poliomyelitis—expending the bulk of these funds in the decade of the 1950s.[7] In its effort to secure an immunizing agent against polio, the National Foundation supported basic and applied research conducted by scores of university-based medical researchers. Its largest project was the 1954–55 field testing of Salk's polio vaccine. Orchestrated by the Foundation, with data analysis overseen by Thomas Francis Jr. at the University of Michigan, the project mobilized the assistance of myriad schools and public health agencies. It involved 1.8 million American children and is still today the largest clinical trial ever conducted in the United States.[8] In the course of such efforts, the Foundation greatly increased the size of its staff and the elaboration of its administrative departments. This included, as suggested in chapter 3, the elaboration of its research division.

The advent of major agencies and organizational divisions devoted to the sponsorship of medical research undoubtedly fostered the systematization of procedures for managing risks of human experiments. Sociologists have long noted a tendency for modern organizations to adopt rationalized structures, policies, and procedures. Writing in the early twentieth century, Max Weber attributed these trends to pressures for efficiency generated by market forces and relations with the state.[9] At midcentury, the major research sponsors displayed many of the features of rational organizations, including management by technically competent personnel, stable divisions of labor, specialized administrative units, and standardized rules and procedures. But pressures for administrative rationality are not the only ones affecting organizational structures and procedures. A recent body of scholarship known as "new institutionalism" suggests that organizations incorporate features of their environment—features with no bearing on work demands or technical efficiency—in an effort to enhance their legitimacy. Organizations that share environments become similar over time in their structures and policies. New institutional theorists identify several isomorphic processes that generate this homogeneity. One involves organizations' importing policies and procedures from rule carriers in their environment, particularly from the professions and the law.[10] The historical record provides ample evidence that this dynamic was operating in sponsors' adoption of procedures for managing the risks of human experiments.

Procedures for Managing Risk

Three procedures were central to the risk-containment strategies of mid-twentieth-century research sponsors: use of consent documents, insurance to compensate for injuries, and scientific-panel oversight of research protocols. Each had roots in the law or contemporary professional practices. Consent had precedents in both legal rulings and professional advocacy. Early in the twentieth century, medical leaders urged that clinical researchers obtain consent from their subjects. In doing so, they were responding to public sentiment and to a series of court rulings issued between 1905 and 1914—particularly the *Schloendorff* decision in 1914—that established basic features of consent to medical treatment in American law.[11] Insurance coverage for researchers also had legal antecedents. Changes in the interpretation of tort law during the 1930s inaugurated widespread use of liability insurance as a means of compensating personal injury cases.[12] Sponsors adapted scientific-panel oversight from the peer review routinely practiced within investigatory communities.

These three measures were not the only ones that sponsors implemented in the pre–World War II period. Some early risk-management measures remained idiosyncratic to particular experiments or sponsors. When Thomas Francis Jr. conducted his 1935 influenza-virus trial, the Rockefeller Institute insisted that he limit his subjects to medical personnel, choose a route of immunization likely to minimize clinical symptoms, and quarantine study participants. These measures did not become routine for other clinical trials. Even those procedures that were relatively widespread were not universally adopted. Insurance coverage was the least well institutionalized of the three measures.[13] Nonetheless, over time, use of consent documents and oversight of hazards by scientific advisory panels become prevalent, routine, and formalized.

Consent

The notion that consent is a vehicle for controlling investigatory hazards rests uneasily with present-day ethical sensibilities. Advocates of human-subjects protections view consent as a matter of moral principle: the individual's prerogative to make decisions about the purposes to which his or her body is put. The *Belmont Report*—a product of the 1974–78 national

bioethics commission—calls this principle "respect for persons."[14] From
the perspective of the *Belmont Report,* consent is a basic right, not a procedure to be used in the interest of professional or organizational politics.
Nonetheless, early-twentieth-century researchers and sponsors routinely
used consent procedures as a means for handling the risks that human experimentation posed for scientific institutions. In doing so, they were following a course advocated by the profession.

Early-twentieth-century medical leaders insisted that consent justified
experiments that would otherwise have been morally unacceptable. William
Osler took this position in a statement made November 20, 1907, before
Britain's Royal Commission on Vivisection. The context of his remarks was
a discussion of Walter Reed's 1900 experiment in which, to discover whether
mosquitoes transmitted yellow fever, researchers deliberately exposed human subjects to infected insects. Osler argued that the experiment was
moral because the subjects were knowledgeable about the dangers of the
procedure and had consented:

> *Commissioner:* We were told by a witness yesterday that, in his opinion,
> to experiment upon man with possible ill result was immoral. Would that
> be your view?
> *Osler:* It is always immoral, without the definite, specific statement
> from the individual himself, with a full knowledge of the circumstances.
> Under these circumstances, any man, I think, is at liberty to submit himself
> to experiments.
> *Commissioner:* Given voluntary consent, you think that entirely changes
> the question of morality or otherwise?
> *Osler:* Entirely.[15]

Researchers consistently invoked consent when confronted with accusations of unjustified human experimentation. For example, William Park and
John Kolmer underscored permission from parents when responding to
questions about the appropriateness of their using newly developed polio
vaccines on children. In the fall of 1934, the U.S. assistant surgeon general,
R. C. Williams, wrote to Park and Kolmer, asking them to respond to press
reports that their polio vaccines were being tested on orphans. Williams was
acting at the behest of First Lady Eleanor Roosevelt, who had received letters
of protest about the use of children in medical experiments. In separate
replies to Williams, Park and Kolmer each insisted that his vaccine was safe.
Before inoculating children, the researchers had tested the preparations on
animals and on members of their own investigatory teams. Kolmer had first

vaccinated his own two youngsters. Most important, the scientists had obtained consent from the children's parents before proceeding. Park's letter to the assistant surgeon general concluded:

> I am sure that when you inform Mrs. Roosevelt of these facts, she will realize that we would not think of doing anything to children which we felt would be harmful to them and that we are not doing it without the *consent of their parents*.[16]

In this instance, as in others, invoking the consent of subjects or their guardians ended accusations of inappropriate human experimentation.

If such incidents reveal that the consent of subjects or their guardians in fact served to mollify critics, social science literature on risk helps to explain why consent would have this impact. Scholars in the field of risk perception have explored public tolerance for technological hazards—airplane accidents, nuclear accidents, toxic waste spills, and the like. Among their findings is that acceptance of technological risk is much greater when hazards are seen as freely chosen rather than imposed. We demand much higher levels of safety for commercial aviation, an indispensable means of travel for the public at large, than for private aviation, where assumption of greater risk is seen as the deliberate choice of small-plane owners. As Chauncey Starr remarks, "We are loath to let others do unto us what we would happily do to ourselves." Starr compared mortality rates associated with a variety of common technological hazards—some voluntary and some involuntary. On this basis, he estimates that "the public is willing to accept 'voluntary' risks roughly 1000 times greater than 'involuntary' risks."[17] Although Starr was examining risk acceptability in the 1960s, his remarks appear applicable also to popular sentiment about medical-research hazards during the first half the century. Indeed, the perceived voluntariness of risk has long been important to public attitudes about hazardous medical interventions.

Early Pressures for Consent

Early-twentieth-century scientific leaders exhorted medical researchers to obtain subjects' consent when conducting experiments. In doing so they were responding to at least two developments: court rulings issued between 1905 and 1914 elaborating the necessity for consent to surgical treatment and the contemporary antivivisection movement, which objected to human as well as animal experimentation. As described in chapter 1, during the early decades of the twentieth century, activists secured coverage of reputed medical-research abuses in the popular press and pushed for bills in both Congress and state legislatures to control the conduct of clinical research. A goal of this legislation was, in the words of one movement spokesman, to ensure that "no experiment . . . be conducted on any . . . human being without his intelligent written consent."[18] Activists triggered widespread public concern about the conduct of human experiments and won considerable support for their legislative goals from the American middle and professional classes. The medical-research community took the threat of legislative controls very seriously.[19]

Professional leaders took a variety of actions to allay public concerns. As discussed in earlier chapters, the AMA established the Council for the Defense of Medical Research in 1908 to coordinate efforts to blunt the impact of antivivisectionism. During the 1910s, physiologist Walter Cannon, the council's head, lobbied informally within the profession for the adoption of consent procedures by medical researchers. Cannon urged that medical journals, when reporting use of a novel medical treatment, require authors to state that the patients or their guardians were fully aware of and consented to the intervention. Cannon contacted medical laboratories recommending that consent be obtained when researchers were conducting deliberate experiments.[20] When arguing for these policies, he invoked both public opinion and the law. In an editorial appearing in *JAMA* in 1916, Cannon wrote:

> There is no more primitive and fundamental right which any individual possesses than that of controlling the uses to which his own body is put. . . . The lay public is perfectly clear about it. . . . And the law, as an expression of public conscience, declares that deliberate injury done to the body of another is an assault, and provides severe punishment for it.[21]

Cannon's wording echoed the rationale for consent to surgical treatment in a contemporary court ruling. Justice Benjamin Cardozo wrote in his decision in the *Schloendorff* case:

> Every human being of adult years and sound mind has the right to determine what shall be done with his own body; and a surgeon who performs an operation without his patient's consent commits an assault, for which he is liable in damages.[22]

Both law and public sentiment prescribed consent to human experimentation, albeit with little guidance as to what form that consent should assume.

Public attitudes about consent affected not only scientists and sponsors, but also the institutions that opened their doors to medical researchers: prisons, long-term-care hospitals, and homes for disabled children. Managers of custodial facilities providing access to human subjects initiated use of some of the earliest consent statements. Jon Harkness examined medical experimentation in American penal institutions and found that "players involved in prison research accepted the need for obtaining consent as obvious, even as early as 1915."[23] Central among these players were institutional directors and the state agencies that oversaw prison management. My exploration of vaccine trials conducted in custodial facilities for children reveals a similar set of assumptions. Joseph Stokes Jr.—the University of Pennsylvania researcher discussed in earlier chapters—tested newly developed influenza and measles vaccines at children's facilities across New Jersey and eastern Pennsylvania during the late 1930s and 1940s. The directors of these institutions viewed the consent of parents as mandatory, particularly for initial tests of a vaccine's safety and therapeutic value.[24]

Arrangements for obtaining consent were central to Stokes's negotiations with children's facilities for access to subjects. The realities of institutional politics made consent procedures necessary. Superintendents of private institutions reported to boards of trustees and other oversight bodies. Heads of public institutions were accountable to state agencies, political appointees, and ultimately the public. Managers of both public and private facilities worried that harm to a child would trigger condemnation of the decision to allow medical experimentation within the institution. Administrators viewed the consent of parents as protection from the threat of such criticism. The correspondence between Stokes and James S. Dean, a physician and superintendent of Pennhurst State School, illustrates this dynamic. Stokes approached Dean about testing a measles vaccine at Pennhurst. In a letter dated June 20, 1941, Dean apprised Stokes of an exchange that he had had with William C. Sandy, director of Pennsylvania's Bureau of Mental Health, under whose aegis the facility operated:

> Dr. Sandy stated that it was a source of great satisfaction to him to learn of your interest in our patients at Pennhurst and in the problems they present. Dr. Sandy pointed out, however, that since we are a public institution, we should exercise every possible precaution to avoid criticism or hazard of an infection. He also pointed out that certain individuals might quite erroneously misinterpret some intercurrent disease as having been attributable to one of the inoculations. I personally feel that this might be circumvented by securing individual permissions from parents or guardians.[25]

Interestingly, Stokes's correspondence reveals that it was often the institutional director, not the research team, who arranged for parental approval.[26] When this was the case, documentation of parental consent was part of the institution's records rather than the researchers'.

Sponsors' Requirements for Written Consent

In the 1940s and 1950s, organizational sponsors of clinical research were requiring written consent statements with increasing regularity. Instances of sponsor-initiated consent documents in earlier decades can certainly be found. As described in chapter 3, when the Board of Scientific Directors at the Rockefeller Institute allowed Thomas Francis Jr. to proceed with his influenza-inoculation experiment in 1935, it developed an elaborate consent document for use in the trial. But it was unusual for the Institute to be supporting a clinical experiment—its principal focus was laboratory research—and drafting consent documents was not standard procedure. In contrast, at the CMR and AEB, the requirement of written consent statements was routine where experiments were considered hazardous. In October of 1942, CMR chairman Alfred N. Richards articulated what would be that agency's policy on the matter:

> When any risks are involved, volunteers only should be utilized as subjects, and these only after the risks have been fully explained and after signed statements have been obtained which shall provide that the volunteer offered his services with full knowledge.[27]

Records of the AEB indicate that it also considered written consent standard procedure for hazardous experiments. The papers of Stokes, who headed the AEB Commission on Measles and Mumps during World War II, include numerous AEB-initiated consent documents dating from the mid-1940s. By the early 1950s, the National Foundation was requiring researchers working under its auspices to obtain written consent when conducting initial trials of new polio vaccines. The Foundation's research division gave directions to both Jonas Salk and Albert Sabin on the wording of consent documents used in early tests of their immunizing agents.[28]

At all of these agencies—the Rockefeller Institute, the CMR, the AEB, and the National Foundation—concern with legal liability was an impetus for written consent documents. Quite frequently in the late 1930s, 1940s, and 1950s, sponsors consulted lawyers about the need for and wording of these documents. Furthermore, many consent statements from this period include a waiver of claims to compensation for research-related injuries. Documents with waiver clauses begin with a description of the experiment being conducted and an affirmation of the subject's willingness to participate. The texts then state that the subject releases scientists and sponsors from legal liability for any harm that might result from his or her participation in the study. The Rockefeller Institute consent form for Francis's influenza-inoculation experiment included a waiver provision drafted by legal counsel. It read in part:

> I hereby assume all risk of personal injury whether due to negligence or otherwise resulting from the introduction or introductions of such virus into my body . . . [and I hereby] release and discharge said Institute, and its successors, and everyone associated or connected with or employed by it or them, from any and all liability, claims or demands whether for negligence or otherwise.[29]

The CMR and AEB routinely included waiver provisions in their consent documents. Richards's policy at the CMR stipulated that consent documents used in hazardous experiments state that the subject's "claims for damages have been waived." The wording of one AEB waiver clause exempted the agency and researchers from liability for "any ill effects, sickness, temporary or permanent disability, or death that might result" as a result of the experiments.[30]

Not all midcentury sponsors included waiver provisions in their consent documents. The National Foundation made an effort to avoid such clauses.[31] The Foundation's concern with public relations shaped its preference about waiver provisions. Dependent upon charitable contributions to support its polio-vaccine efforts, the National Foundation was very sensitive about its image. It was also aware of the public relations value of consent documents. The Foundation treated consent statements not only as legal documents but also as tools for facilitating the recruitment of subjects. In 1953, when planning for the national field trial of Jonas Salk's polio vaccine, the Foundation sought out reactions from a variety of commentators when drafting the parental-consent form. The advice it received was to avoid legalism and make consent statements responsive to the concerns of the subjects' parents.[32]

But on at least one occasion, the National Foundation had its name included in a waiver clause. In 1955, when Albert Sabin conducted initial human tests of live polio strains at the Chillicothe Federal Reformatory, he used a consent form that released the National Foundation, the Children's

Hospital Research Foundation at the University of Cincinnati, the U.S. Bureau of Prisons, and all personnel associated with these institutions from liability for injury. Initially, the National Foundation's legal department told Sabin to leave the Foundation's name out of the consent document. It then reversed its position. Stephen Ryan, the organization's general counsel, told Sabin that, "it was the National Foundation's insurer that was desirous of having the Foundation's name in the consent form."[33]

Neither early court rulings nor professional advocacy specified the form that consent to human experimentation should assume. Yet by midcentury, consent statements used by major sponsors had substantial similarities. These documents named the subject, researchers, and sponsors. They mentioned the purpose of the study and the nature of the intervention being tested. Many included waivers of the subject's claims to compensation for injury. Apart from types of mishaps alluded to in waiver clauses, consent statements from the middle decades of the century included little or no elaboration of the likely risks entailed in a human experiment. The documents did, however, provide written affirmation that the subject's participation in the research was voluntary.

Insurance

Although insurance was the least prevalent of the three measures for handling research risks, archival documents reveal that, in the early 1940s, some scientists and sponsors were discussing the purchase of commercial insurance for subjects who might be injured in a hazardous medical experiment. Insurance was only one available provision for subjects sickened in the course of research. On some occasions, sponsors undertook medical treatment of subjects. The consent documents for several AEB-sponsored experiments include the statement that the board would assume responsibility for treating acute illnesses associated with the research.[34] Such provisions for short-term medical care notwithstanding, researchers sought insurance coverage for subjects, paid for by their organizational sponsor.

Scientists receiving AEB and CMR funding, as well as those serving on agency oversight boards, made periodic efforts to secure insurance coverage for human subjects. Documents reveal that these federal agencies had three responses. First, officials viewed the cost of insurance for subjects—whether life, accident, medical, or disability coverage—to be prohibitively expensive. Second, in the hands of government lawyers—to whom such issues were referred—questions about insurance coverage for subjects were translated into questions about the liability of researchers, their employers, and the U.S. government. If insurance was to be purchased, it would be coverage for institutions and investigators, not for research subjects. Federal contracts apparently sometimes allowed for liability coverage for scientists. For example, in 1942, the CMR authorized an experiment testing methods for preventing and curing gonorrhea that involved deliberately infecting prison inmates with the disease. When discussing the potential legal liability associated with the experiment, Richards wrote that "arrangements can be made whereby both [researchers] and the Institution can be protected by insurance."[35] But the government's third and preferred solution was not to provide insurance for researchers, much less for subjects, but rather to rely on the indemnification of federal contractors and on waiver provisions included in consent statements.

This preference is clear from Jon Harkness's account of a hazardous CMR experiment, conducted in 1942, involving human testing of bovine blood plasma. CMR leaders had requested government payment for insurance for subjects in the trial. The OSRD's chief attorney, who was handling the matter, reported that the insurance carrier he had consulted was unwilling to assume coverage for subjects. In the end, OSRD lawyers arranged indemnification for the university contracting to conduct the study.[36] A similar course of events unfolded in 1947, when Stokes asked the AEB about reimbursement for disability insurance for inmates in a New Jersey state prison who were serving as subjects in risk-laden hepatitis experiments. The AEB's legal department detailed its position in a letter to its scientific division:

> The question of reimbursing the contractor for payment of the premium on a disability policy on a prisoner during the experiment, was submitted to the Contract Insurance Branch, Office of the Chief of Finance. They advised that there was no authority for taking out such a policy and that it would not be approved. They further stated that they discussed the question of such coverage with the private underwriter and were advised that the cost would be prohibitive.

The letter continues:

> This office, accordingly, recommends that Dr. Stokes be advised to protect himself, the State of New Jersey, and the Government, by means of the usual waiver.[37]

If federal agencies resisted providing insurance for subjects or researchers, by the 1950s, the National Foundation was requiring it. When Albert Sabin was preparing to test his live-polio vaccine at Chillicothe prison, he received a directive from the Foundation advising him of the necessity for insurance coverage. The communication cited precedence: "When Doctor Howe carried out his first series of experiments [with formalin-treated polio strains] on six children in Baltimore, special accident and health insurance policies were taken out. Similar arrangements were also made in the case of Doctor Salk."[38] The National Foundation quickly extended the policy to cover all the researchers it funded.[39] Policy directives referring to "accident and health insurance" suggest that the Foundation was providing coverage for both investigators and subjects. Although I found no corroborating evidence concerning insurance for subjects, evidence of insurance for researchers is clear. In January of 1955, Sabin reported using National Foundation funds to purchase "liability and malpractice insurance" for himself and the Children's Hospital Research Foundation.[40]

At midcentury, waiver provisions and insurance for researchers were alternative strategies for protecting scientists and sponsors from legal liability for research injuries. Even while waiver provisions were used by major research sponsors, opinion was weighted against them. The clauses were problematic in part because many legal advisors considered waivers unlikely to hold up to legal challenge.[41] Furthermore, release clauses were antithetical to the research community's efforts to sustain public trust in the conduct of medical experiments. Irving Ladimer commented on the moral status of waiver provisions in a 1954 article on legal and ethical aspects of human experimentation:

> The inclusion of [a waiver] provision would be considered ethically unacceptable to a profession concerned with safeguarding health and might cast suspicion on any project. Commercial insurance coverage and provision of medical care for consequences directly relating to the project are methods observed by responsible organizations.[42]

If waiver provisions were considered morally suspect, insurance was never fully established either.[43] Some scientists and policy advocates considered provisions for compensating injury to be the responsible course to take in the face of investigatory hazards. But in the arena of medical research, written consent, not insurance for research or subjects, would become sponsors' primary response to the potential of liability for human injury.

Advisory-Panel Oversight

Scientific advisory boards were virtually universal among the major mid-century sponsors of medical research. These panels had primary functions other than monitoring experimental hazards. They often provided scientific direction to the organization's research efforts and made recommendations about project funding. But when a particularly hazardous study was under consideration or when other moral issues arose, the boards stepped in. In chapter 3, I described two examples of this pattern from the mid-1930s. At the Rockefeller Institute, the Board of Scientific Directors closely monitored Francis's 1935 influenza-inoculation experiment. Directors were available while the experiment was ongoing, ready to respond if a situation unfolded requiring medical or political management. At the President's Birthday Ball Commission (PBBC)—later the National Foundation—the scientific advisory board addressed risks of continued use of the Park-Brodie polio vaccine and terminated distribution of the immunizing agent when serious concerns arose about the preparation's safety.

Sponsors differed in how they constituted their advisory boards and the extent to which board members had diverse or overlapping competencies. The composition of the CMR covered a wide range of medical fields, but the agency also drew on committees within the National Research Council's medical-science division that had specialized competencies. The AEB had an oversight board with broad competencies in epidemic illnesses, as well as commissions focused on delimited fields of infectious disease. At the AEB, these commissions not only oversaw project support, they were also actively engaged in research. While scientific panels for military agencies addressed issues raised by experiments understood to be problematic, I found no evidence that these agencies instituted procedures for routinely scrutinizing risks of human experiments conducted under their sponsorship.

When NIH set up procedures for reviewing clinical experiments conducted by in-house scientists, it also limited oversight to experiments understood to be problematic. NIH initiated its policy in 1953, with the opening of its hospital. Agency guidelines from that year mandated group review of experimental procedures "deviating from accepted medical practice or involving unusual hazard."[44] The hospital's medical board established the Clinical Research Committee (CRC) to discuss proposals for particularly hazardous human research. Agency policy also directed each NIH institute to create a committee to evaluate especially risky protocols and refer unsolved problems to the CRC.

The National Foundation had a fully developed system for scientific-

panel oversight of ongoing polio research. In the early 1950s, the Foundation required advisory-panel approval of all experiments involving human
testing. By then, the Foundation had several standing committees of scientific experts. This included the Committee on Immunization, composed
of scientists actively engaged in polio-vaccine development. Harry Weaver,
the Foundation's director of research through September 1953, described
the organization's peer-review policy to Irving Ladimer, who in April of that
year was compiling information about oversight of human experimentation
for NIH. Ladimer reported:

> Dr. Weaver emphasized that . . . obtaining appropriate group consideration
> is of utmost importance. Whereas investigators have no objection to dis-
> cussing their proposals before a body of peers they are highly individualis-
> tic and not always disinterested in a matter of personal importance. Accord-
> ingly, as a matter of policy, the Foundation has encouraged scientists and
> investigators to discuss their propositions thoroughly under the observa-
> tions of an informed impartial group. Final decision for recommending ac-
> tion . . . rests with the impartial group.[45]

In fact, the Foundation's leadership found many polio researchers to be far
from impartial. Members of the Committee on Immunization disagreed
sharply over the preferability of a killed vaccine like Salk's or an attenuated
live vaccine like Sabin's. In part for this reason, in May of 1953, the Foundation created a smaller panel, the Vaccine Advisory Committee, composed of
several polio virologists and a number of public health experts, to oversee
immunization trials.[46] It was the Vaccine Advisory Committee, along with
the Foundation's research division, that reviewed Sabin's plan to undertake
human trials of live polio strains at Chillicothe.[47]

In 1966, NIH would mandate peer review of the human-subjects research it supported through its external grants program. These review bodies would be located not within NIH, but rather at the institutions receiving
federal aid. Until NIH issued this protocol-review policy, universities and
hospitals were not major players in oversight of human experimentation.
Some universities did offer advice to faculty regarding the conduct of clinical research. In 1962, a number of departments of medicine reported that
they provided advisory review of human-subjects protocols. In addition, a
handful of academic institutions had committees offering optional review of
proposals for clinical research. The University of Washington created such a
body in 1946. Johns Hopkins University did so in 1949.[48] But through the
mid-1960s, the center of gravity of human-subjects oversight was with the

organizations sponsoring medical research, not the institutions employing scientists.

The Dynamics of Standardization

In the 1940s and 1950s, major sponsors of clinical research in the United States differed somewhat in their approaches to managing the hazards of human experiments. Points of divergence included use of waiver clauses in consent documents and policies toward insurance for researchers and subjects. Sponsors varied also in how they constituted scientific panels—whether members had broad or specialized competencies—and in the regularity with which these bodies addressed hazards entailed in research protocols. But virtually all major sponsors had measures for containing risk, and these included use of written consent documents and access to scientific advisory boards capable of evaluating investigatory hazards. By midcentury, risk-containment measures were routine and formalized, with substantial similarities across research sponsors. Scientists came to see written consent and advisory-panel review as expected, if not universal, requirements of receiving support for the conduct of human experiments.

Thus far I have argued that three processes helped foster a rudimentary system for containing the risks of human experiments. As outlined above, these included the advent of large-scale research sponsors; their tendency to institute rational procedures and policies; and their propensity to import structures and procedures from their environment, particularly from the professions and the law. Each of the risk-management measures prevalent among midcentury sponsors had precedents in legal rulings and the practices of the scientific community. This pattern is consistent with the predictions of new institutional theory, which suggests that organizations become similar over time in part by incorporating features from their environment. But emulation of rule carriers was not the only isomorphic process that shaped sponsors' risk-management strategies. In response to uncertainty about how to comply with existing law, sponsors also imitated the practices of other sponsors.[49]

Recent socio-legal scholarship emphasizes that the law bearing on organizational conduct is often not a clear-cut, known entity. Rather, legal precedents are ambiguous, and notions about what constitutes conformity to the law are, to a considerable degree, socially constructed. Sociologists who adopt this perspective argue that, faced with ambiguity in the law, organizations look to other organizations for clues to how to satisfy legal requirements. Organizations, they suggest, come to collective understandings of what constitutes conformity to the law. Professionals play a key role in this process, by both defining the meaning of legal compliance and promoting these definitions through network links among practitioners and organizations.[50] Historical records on the conduct of clinical research suggest that such dynamics were at work during the first half of the century among the sponsors of human experiments, particularly regarding the use of consent documents.

At midcentury, liability for injuries to human subjects fell into a gray area of the law. William Curran notes that it was not until 1935 that American courts addressed deliberate human experimentation. Earlier rulings that had used the term "medical experiment" referred, not to a planned scientific activity, but, rather, to a deviation from standard medical practice, a transgression that left the clinician open to suit for malpractice.[51] The Michigan Supreme Court issued one of the first American legal opinions commenting explicitly on deliberate experimentation. The case was *Fortner v. Koch* in 1935. While the case did not itself involve medical research, the decision included the following statement:

> We recognize the fact that, if the general practice of medicine and surgery is to progress, there must be a certain amount of experimentation carried on; but such experiments must be done with the knowledge and consent of the patient or those responsible for him, and must not vary too radically from the accepted method of procedure.[52]

This ruling opened the possibility of a legitimate arena for human experimentation so long as the researcher obtained consent and the novel intervention remained within the bounds of reasonableness. It did not specify what evidence of consent was sufficient to protect researchers and sponsors from legal liability. Nor did it indicate the acceptable limits of deviation from standard practice. The decision implied that injury from nontherapeutic experimentation might be handled severely. Thus *Fortner v. Koch* by no means ended uncertainty about the legal status of human experimentation.

Between the mid-1930s and mid-1950s, managers of virtually all of the major sponsors of medical research discussed the possibility of legal action in the event of a research accident.[53] Concern about legal liability remained in the postwar years. The author of a 1954 article on ethical and legal issues in human experimentation spoke of an "imminent possibility of litigation" for research injuries.[54] But if the perceived threat of legal action was clear, the reality of lawsuits was not. Curran examined law pertaining to human experimentation and found "no reported court actions involving liability issues or criminal actions against research organizations or personnel" through the late 1960s.[55]

Faced with ambiguity about legal requirements for avoiding or minimizing liability for research injuries, sponsors emulated the consent practices of other sponsors.[56] Scientists and sponsors regularly solicited consent forms from other institutions and drew on these models when drafting their own documents. While examining materials at archival repositories, I found that folders containing an investigator's consent statements very often included copies of statements used by other researchers. The Rockefeller Institute secured a copy of the consent form used in an experiment at Columbia-Presbyterian Hospital when developing the statement to be used in Francis's 1935 influenza trial. Alfred Dochez, a Columbia-Presbyterian physician who sat on the Institute's scientific board, provided this document. Stokes and Salk traded consent forms in November of 1952, when Stokes was preparing to conduct human tests with variants of Salk's killed-polio vaccine. The researchers sent copies of the exchanged documents, along with related correspondence, to Harry Weaver at the National Foundation.[57] Before undertaking his polio-vaccine trial at Chillicothe in 1955, Sabin told the National Foundation's legal department that he had "adapted the form previously used by the National Institutes of Health in their studies on respiratory infections in volunteers at Chillicothe." A copy of the NIH form is in Sabin's files.[58]

Whether the sharing of consent statements was initiated by the researcher or the sponsor, medical scientists were the conduits for these exchanges. Trading consent forms was part of a much broader pattern of interactions among contemporary researchers. As discussed in chapter 2, networks of medical investigators routinely shared biological materials, information about laboratory techniques, and news of research findings prior to publication. The wording of consent documents was one more resource traded freely through colleague networks.

Enabling Risk-Laden Research

The emerging system for managing clinical-research hazards by no means translated into fewer dangerous human experiments. Indeed, as major sponsors were instituting procedures for managing risks, some were also pursuing extremely risk-laden nontherapeutic experiments. Hazardous studies conducted at midcentury included vaccine trials using what researchers refer to as "challenge" procedures. In these experiments, researchers inoculated a group of subjects with an experimental vaccine, designating another group as controls. After a brief interim, investigators deliberately exposed both vaccinated and unvaccinated subjects to the unmodified pathogen. Researchers fully expected that many subjects—typically inmates of custodial institutions—would contract the disease to which they were exposed. During the 1940s and 1950s, the AEB sponsored numerous challenge experiments testing vaccines against influenza and measles. These trials allowed researchers to assess with great speed the short-term effectiveness of an immunizing agent. Federal agencies sponsored other types of studies where researchers deliberately sickened human subjects. As already mentioned, the CMR approved an experiment giving gonorrhea to prison inmates for the purpose of testing methods for prophylaxis and treatment. The AEB sponsored other studies in which researchers purposefully infected subjects with serious infectious diseases, including dengue fever and hepatitis, for which no animal models were available.[59] The aim of these experiments was to discover the means of transmission, to identify disease strains, and, ultimately, to find methods for treatment and prevention.

A fundamental irony about sponsors' risk-management strategies is that they served to enable the conduct of extremely dangerous nontherapeutic experiments. Among the insights of new institutionalism is that, when organizations adopt legitimizing features from their environment, they often do so in form rather than substance. Imported procedures and policies symbolize the organization's conformity to the expectations of the broader society but may have little to with how the organization actually goes about performing its work.[60] The historical record suggests that, at midcentury, sponsors' implementation of consent was largely ceremonial. Written consent served to invoke a social ideal—the subject's right to decide about the uses to which his or her body was put—but institutions often paid scant attention to the substance of that ideal.

In the early decades of the twentieth century, the research community looked to common law as a representation of cultural values. Walter Cannon pointed to contemporary legal rulings when urging clinical researchers to obtain the consent of their subjects. In doing so, he made explicit reference to the law as "an expression of public conscience."[61] Initially, scientists and organizations involved in clinical research—including custodial facilities providing access to subjects—viewed consent as a means for conforming to social prescriptions and for diffusing public criticism. But by the 1940s, major sponsors were looking to the law less as an exemplar of values than as a source of information on how to avoid legal sanctions. Thus, consent increasingly became a way for sponsors to buffer themselves from the damaging consequences of research-induced human injury. Implemented in this manner, consent not only fell short of protecting subjects, but may actually have allowed sponsors to support experiments involving levels of risk higher than they might otherwise have been willing to assume.

Meanwhile, the cultural ethos of wartime and postwar America fostered permissiveness toward experimental hazards. The prevailing ideology placed sacrifice for the common good above the individual's well-being and rights. David Rothman has commented on the utilitarianism that permeated the research community during the 1940s and 1950s.[62] War Department agencies emphasized that the outcome of human experimentation would aid in the nation's defense. They calculated that the benefits to society of hazardous but rigorously conducted research outweighed the risks to human subjects. An attitude of permissiveness toward very risky experiments affected not only these federal agencies but other sponsors as well.

Research sponsors did not simply rely on contemporary ideological currents to create public tolerance for risk-laden human experiments. They actively generated rhetoric and imagery designed to shape perceptions of the acceptability of hazardous experiments. The sponsoring organizations constructed socially palatable images of human experimentation and presented them to the press and public. In doing so, sponsors were following the lead of the professional community.

A Language of Public Good

I have commented several times on efforts by the early-twentieth-century professional leaders to neutralize criticism of investigatory practices leveled by antivivisection activists. Walter Cannon, head of the AMA's Council for the Defense of Medical Research from 1908 through 1926, lobbied newspaper editors and publishers in an effort to influence the tenor of articles on human experiments. The council created a press bureau to assist in these efforts.[63] Accounts in the popular press were a problem, in part because, consistent with the antivivisectionist sympathies of is owner, the Hearst newspaper chain routinely carried stories about investigatory practices it found objectionable.[64] One of the scientific community's early strategies for protecting its public image was to avoid presentations of human experimentation in professional journals—antivivisectionists routinely scanned these publications—that might trigger negative publicity. From the 1920s through the 1940s, Peyton Rous, then editor of the *Journal of Experimental Medicine,* reviewed submissions with an eye toward avoiding complaints from activists. On at least one occasion, he declined to publish an article that he thought might provoke protest.[65] Rous asked other authors to make changes in the title or content of their papers. He was especially alert to the language used in describing human experiments. Rous advised authors to substitute "test" for "experiment," and to refer to research subjects as "volunteers."[66]

Meanwhile, in commentary directed to outside audiences, scientific leaders emphasized preventive and therapeutic gains resulting from clinical experiments. Laboratory medicine could generate breakthroughs in disease eradication, but human testing was indispensable for realizing this progress. During World War II and the immediate postwar years, public discourse incorporated a new set of metaphors about clinical research. The laboratory was a battlefield, and both researchers and subjects were combatants in the fight against disease. In this period, descriptions of medical research appearing in the popular press invoked courage, heroism, and sacrifice for the common good. Accounts alluded to laudable motivations on the part of researchers and subjects. The research community promoted this rhetoric.[67]

By midcentury, research sponsors were also participating in the public construction of human experimentation. In the 1940s, the AEB intervened with reporters and editors to shape coverage of risk-laden human experiments. Colonel Stanhope Bayne-Jones, the physician-researcher within the Office of the Army Surgeon General who served as the AEB's executive secretary, routinely monitored press accounts of board-sponsored research. Bayne-Jones corresponded with the science editor of the *New York Times,* sending reprints and complimenting the paper on reportage that he judged to be "fair and balanced." On numerous occasions, Bayne-Jones arranged release of information to the press in exchange for editorial control over resulting articles. He would instruct board-funded researchers to cooperate with a reporter if the newspaper in question agreed to submit stories to the Office of the Army Surgeon General for clearance. He then negotiated with editors over the tone and content of articles.

Bayne-Jones's correspondence with G. D. Fairbairn, an editor at the *Philadelphia Evening Bulletin,* illustrates this strategy. In February 1945, Fairbairn wrote to Bayne-Jones requesting cooperation in preparation of a feature article on what Fairbairn referred to as the the "guinea pigs" in the "jaundice experiments on the University of Pennsylvania campus." Bayne-Jones responded: "Permission is granted for the preparation of this article provided the article is submitted to me for clearance through the Technical Information Division of The Surgeon General's Office prior to publication." The colonel continued:

It is hoped that in the preparation of this story the writer will maintain a moderate tone, and that exaggeration of the facts will be avoided. May I suggest that the term "guinea pigs" for these *volunteers* is undignified, hackneyed, threadbare and hardly appropriate. I hope you can find a more fitting term for these men.[68]

Bayne-Jones sought both use of the term "volunteers" and a laudatory account of the motivations of those participating in the research—both subjects and scientists.

Nowhere was the public relations of science more adept than at the National Foundation, whose managers viewed the social legitimacy of its research programs as a matter of crucial importance.[69] Early in the 1940s, the Foundation hired a consultant in scientific public relations. His work included handling press releases, drafting popularized accounts of Foundation research projects for magazines and news syndicates, and interacting with science writers. In the mid-1940s, an in-house professional relations bureau took over the job of disseminating information about the Foundation's research program. Meanwhile the organization established a dedicated public relations department, and between 1944 and 1952, the number of professional staff assigned to this department grew from one person to twelve.[70]

With its attention to popular attitudes and expertise in public relations, the National Foundation demonstrated exceptional ingenuity in constructing palatable imagery of human experimentation. When planning the field trial of Salk's polio vaccine, which took place in 1954–55, the Foundation launched a campaign to promote public participation in the clinical experiment. The organization worded its consent forms so that parents were not granting permission to have their children be part of a medical experiment but, rather, were requesting that their youngsters be included in a unique opportunity. The consent statement bore the title "Parental Request for Participation of Child." It read, in part: "I hereby request that my child . . . be permitted to participate." Children receiving vaccinations were not "subjects" or even "volunteers," but "polio pioneers."[71] The National Foundation skillfully integrated metaphors of American initiative and heroism into popular discourse on its polio-vaccine trials.

Professional leaders and organizational managers viewed public support as necessary to the sustained conduct of human experiments. Without popular support, many research institutions would have difficulty attracting resources, and the scientific community would be vulnerable to pressures for legislative control of human and animal research. Public endorsement was crucial for two other reasons as well. First, it was indispensable to the recruitment of research subjects. Directors of institutions providing access to subjects were alert to social attitudes concerning the propriety of human experimentation taking place within their doors. The superintendent of one children's facility wrote to Stokes, who sought access for a measles-vaccine experiment: "I am eager to cooperate with you because I realize that this piece of work will not just aid our children but will be of great benefit to all children."[72] It was the widespread belief that such experiments were in the common good that allowed scientists to conduct human trials in custodial facilities during the early and middle decades of the twentieth century.

Second, public sentiment would determine the extent to which an investigatory accident would prove damaging to the organization sponsoring the research. In 1942, when the CMR was considering the experiment that involved infecting prison inmates with gonorrhea, OSRD managers consulted attorneys. At issue was whether the consent of subjects would protect the agency from liability in the event of legal suit. The OSRD's own attorney took the position that the outcome of legal action would be "a question of 'public policy'—whether the public welfare favors it." In this view, a court decision would favor the agency because "when a country is at war . . . and [gonorrhea] is taking a terrific toll of the Armed Forces . . . the nation should be allowed to freely accept such voluntary sacrifices by its citizens."[73] In short, the disposition of a legal suit would ultimately rest upon public attitudes.

Shaping Public Accounts of Medical Research

After World War II, the medical-research community redoubled its effort at public persuasion, setting out to enlighten the press—and through it the public—about the methods and rationale for human and animal experiments. In 1946, academic leaders created a new organization, the National Society for Medical Research (NSMR). The society sent newsletters to science writers and offered a weekly research report to local radio stations. It distributed an abundance of material for popular consumption on both clinical and laboratory research. Medical investigators' openness about methods of clinical research was consistent with strategies used by other scientific communities that launched public relations campaigns after the war to enhance popular appreciation of science.[74]

Medical researchers and their sponsors have not been alone in their efforts to shape public perceptions and attitudes about technological hazards. Scholarship on risk shows that, at least since the second half of the twentieth century, a range of organizations implementing potentially hazardous technologies have sought to affect public sentiment and policy. With increasing regularity, these organizations have employed professional analysts to calculate the benefits of risky endeavors and the probabilities for accidents or failure. When invoked in policy debates, such analyses serve to normalize risk. After examining contingency plans for technological disasters and accidents—plans for oil spills, nuclear power plant meltdowns, and nuclear attacks—Lee Clarke concluded that these plans are symbolic in character and formulated as tools for political persuasion.[75]

Social science literature points to several factors encouraging organizations that apply modern technologies to undertake efforts at public persuasion: perceptions of technological hazards are highly malleable; what constitutes acceptable risk is socially constructed; and the public's comfort with hazards rests in large measure on its trust in the institutions that make determinative judgments about risk assumption. Moreover, shifting cultural and ideological currents affect notions about risk acceptability.[76] My analysis suggests that other dynamics operate as well. Because public responses to hazards affect whether risk assumption will be a liability to organizations, shaping public perceptions is a way to reduce organizational uncertainty. But the success of this strategy rests on the institutional community's ability to mobilize dominant cultural symbols and to counteract imagery generated by regulatory movements. The media has been a crucial location for these struggles.[77]

Ironies of Organizational Oversight

Research sponsors have capabilities for controlling investigatory risk not available to loosely constituted colleague networks. Organizations can mobilize the expertise of scientific specialists to evaluate and monitor the dangers of human research. They can impose formal procedures to contain hazards and terminate or decline funding for excessively risky studies. Often, however, organizations' potential for exercising judicious oversight is not fully realized.

A two-sided picture of medical-research oversight in America emerges from the historical records of the 1940s and 1950s. Several powerful organizations began to construct a formal and homogenous system for managing research hazards. They created scientific advisory panels to review investigatory protocols, required use of written consent documents, and sometimes provided scientists with insurance that would compensate for research injuries. However, these measures did not mean that human subjects were protected. While contemporary sponsors varied in their level of tolerance for hazards, two federal agencies that supported university-based medical researchers embarked on some of the most dangerous human experiments conducted in the nation's history. It was precisely when risks were most grave that leaders at the wartime AEB and CMR took most care to implement procedures for containing the potential consequences of risk assumption. The measures they adopted—advisory-panel oversight, liability insurance, and use of written consent with waiver provisions—may have served to normalize hazards, allowing sponsors to proceed with experiments they might otherwise have been more reluctant to pursue.

In accounting for this irony, I have drawn on recent institutional theory, which suggests that, while organizations tend to adopt procedures that signal conformity with social norms, they also tend to implement these measures so that ceremony takes precedence over substantive compliance. But if institutional processes help to explain the normalization of research risks during the 1940s and 1950s, the wartime ethos in America undoubtedly contributed as well. This ethos promoted contributions to the common good even where they involved tremendous individual costs. Patterns in wartime and postwar medical research are a reminder that prevailing cultural currents exert a powerful influence on boundaries between acceptable and unacceptable human experiments. They are a reminder also of the essential malleability of constructions of risk.

5

The Social Nature of Moral Action

Social control of human experimentation in America can be thought of as having three distinct phases. In the first, extending through the early decades of the twentieth century, oversight of medical research was the exclusive purview of communities of scientists that maintained rich traditions for the moral conduct of human experiments. At the core of these traditions was a logic of lesser harms, whereby a hazardous clinical intervention was acceptable if it yielded net benefit and its risks were lower than those of the natural disease. Other features of researchers' informal morality were an insistence on sound scientific work, on animal experiments before human trials, on clinical moratoria until problems generating undue risk were solved in the laboratory, and on self-experimentation. The historical record shows that communities of researchers articulated lesser-harm reasoning as far back as the early eighteenth century. By the second half of the nineteenth century, investigators in emerging fields of laboratory medicine were embracing all features of this informal morality.

The second phase dates to the middle third of the twentieth century. In this period, organizations sponsoring medical research instituted procedures for managing the risks of clinical experiments. Over time, procedures became more routine, formalized, and similar across sponsors. Several processes fostered organizational oversight of human experimentation: the appearance of large-scale research sponsors during and after World War II; the trend toward rationalization typical of modern organizations; the propensity of organizations to import legitimacy-conferring procedures and policies from the professional and legal environment. In adopting risk-management measures, sponsoring organizations were drawing from the practices of the medical-research community and from the interpretation of tort law. The procedures adopted included written consent documents, insurance for researchers, and scientific-panel oversight of investigatory protocols.

In the third phase, beginning in the 1960s, government agencies inaugurated formal regulation of human experimentation. In response to 1962 congressional legislation, the Food and Drug Administration initiated measures for overseeing the clinical testing of experimental medical products. In 1966, the National Institutes of Health (NIH) began requiring that local peer-review committees approve agency-funded human experiments. These provisions notwithstanding, controversy over human-subjects protections grew within both scientific circles and national policy arenas. In 1974, in the face of mounting pressure for further governmental controls, the U.S. Department of Health, Education, and Welfare—later the Department of Health and Human Services (DHHS)—issued NIH policy as federal regulatory code. That year, Congress passed legislation establishing a bioethics panel, the National Commission for the Protection of Human Subjects of Biomedical and Behavioral Research, to recommend additional regulatory provisions. In subsequent decades, federal policymakers revised and augmented standards to be used in research-protocol review. DHHS codes delegate oversight of human-subjects protocols to institutional review boards (IRBs) of organizations that receive federal research funding. Regulatory law directs these boards to pay particular attention to the risks and benefits of proposed experiments and to investigators' plans for securing the voluntary and informed consent of subjects. Government policy since the 1980s has encouraged research institutions to apply oversight codes to all human research—whether federally funded or not.

Some readers may find problematic my contention that a loosely constituted system for overseeing human experiments existed before 1960. If the scientific community observed moral traditions in the conduct of human experiments, how was it possible for researchers to conduct, and much of the scientific community to condone, experiments identified in the 1960s and 1970s as investigatory abuses? Moreover, how could investigators and federal sponsors have justified the nontherapeutic experiments conducted during the 1940s and 1950s that deliberately sickened subjects—experiments not identified in public arenas as research excesses? Scrutiny of historical records makes it clear that pursuit of the types of research repudiated during the 1960s and 1970s went well beyond an occasional incident. Commentary from within the research community corroborates this observation. Harvard anesthesiologist Henry Beecher, a whistle blower from within the scientific community, declared in the mid-1960s that researchers were routinely conducting excessively risky human experiments with little or no benefit for participants. He argued that they were often doing so without subjects' full knowledge or voluntary consent. According to Beecher, these practices were both widespread and endemic to elite circles of medical science.[1] If both indigenous morality and organizational procedures for managing risk were in place, how could scientists have committed investigatory excesses on this scale?

The Changing Cultural Context of Medical Research

I argued in chapter 4 that procedures used by midcentury sponsors for securing consent were, in large measure, ceremonial. Many consent statements used by sponsors during this period included provisions that waived the subject's right to compensation in the event of injury. While symbolizing deference to public sentiments regarding voluntary participation in medical research, these documents served to buffer the organization from damages rather than to protect human subjects. Consent implemented in this manner had the ironic consequence of enabling sponsors to pursue extremely hazardous research. But if ceremonial consent helped foster the conduct of dangerous human experiments during the middle decades of twentieth century, contemporary ideological currents contributed as well.

Moral traditions have enjoined researchers to weigh the hazards of medical interventions against the dangers of natural disease and to ensure that human experiments yield net benefit. Oversight by sponsors has generated procedures for the conduct of clinical trials. But neither moral traditions nor organizational oversight has determined how scientists define risks and benefits or where they draw boundaries between acceptable and unacceptable experiments. For both researchers and sponsors, the culture outside the research community has powerfully shaped constructions of what constitutes justifiable risk.

Decisions about proceeding with hazardous clinical research involve tensions between two competing social goals: the rights and well-being of the individual and the good of society at large. The relative priority of these goals shifts periodically in response to broader ideological currents. Between the 1940s and 1970s, two transitions took place in American cultural

sensibilities that affected notions of appropriate medical risk. The first began with America's entrance into World War II and generated dramatically
increased tolerance for investigatory hazards. The second began with the social activism of the 1960s and triggered pressing concerns about mistreat-
ment of subjects and the rejection of previously accepted standards for investigatory conduct. The emergence of research abuses as a public problem
in the 1960s was the product of a clash between two disparate historical sensibilities: America's wartime and postwar culture that applauded sacrifices
for the common good and the ethos emerging in the 1960s concerned with
the misuse of individuals by those with more power.

During World War II and the Cold War years, a utilitarian ethos domi-
nated medical scientists' stance toward the conduct of human experiments.[2] Social commentators routinely applauded individuals who placed
contributions to the country's war effort before their own interests. A broad
range of citizens were making potentially life-threatening sacrifices in the
national interest. Why should human subjects in medical research be an exception? I have suggested that scientists promoted public acceptance of dangerous clinical research by formulating accounts of human experiments
that incorporated valued cultural symbols. These accounts drew upon imagery of the battlefield and lauded the heroism of those they called volunteers for medical science. The prevailing cultural climate significantly
affected scientists' risk-benefit calculations. When considering the acceptability of human experiments, researchers emphasized expected gains for
medical knowledge and substantially relaxed their observation of lesser-
harm logic when it came to outcomes for subjects. The wartime ethos of
sacrifice for the common good preempted lesser-harm reasoning and justified nontherapeutic research with no benefit for subjects.

The 1960s witnessed a dramatic shift in America's cultural climate. The
priority of common social goals gave way to a dominant concern with ex-
ploitation of the disadvantaged. Radical social movements generalized the
logic of civil rights to a range of other constituencies, including patients, institutionalized populations, and research subjects.[3] In light of this new cultural ethos, risk-laden experiments acceptable during the preceding two
decades could no longer be justified. Policy advocates called for governmental controls and new standards for the conduct of human experiments. They
sought rules compatible with the renewed emphasis on individual rights
and with legal decisions in medical-malpractice cases issued in the late
1950s and 1960s. In these rulings—among them the *Salgo* case in 1957—
the court specified that the patients' self-determination required that consent to medical treatment had to be fully informed.[4] Repudiation of investi-

gatory abuses during the 1960s and 1970s was a feature of political advocacy for regulatory reform. The episodes of research abuse that became most visible in public arenas—experiments conducted at the Jewish Chronic Disease Hospital in Brooklyn; at Willowbrook State School on Staten Island; and at Tuskegee, Alabama—were ones that exemplified scientists' failure to conform to the new standards for consent that policy advocates sought to include in federal regulatory law. These experiments were also ones where researchers drew their subjects from powerless groups: deteriorated elderly patients at the Jewish Chronic Disease Hospital, disabled children at Willowbrook, and impoverished African Americans at Tuskegee.[5]

The Emergence of Government Regulation

A detailed discussion of the creation of federal human-subjects protections is outside the scope of this book. But I will make several observations about government oversight that flow from the preceding analysis. It is clear that the government system incorporated key features of institutionally embedded rules and procedures that preceded it—albeit in modified forms. The core features retained were written consent, peer review of research protocols, and the injunction to weigh risks and benefits when evaluating the appropriateness of human experiments.

At the same time, federal regulatory codes inaugurated substantive changes in the oversight of human experiments. Among these was an overhaul of the rules for consent. I have noted several times that early-twentieth-century researchers considered consent necessary when subjects were healthy and interventions were hazardous. But the need for consent was less clear when subjects were patients and experimental interventions therapeutic in intent.[6] Ambiguities in the informal rules left considerable room for the influence of both investigators' moral inclinations and the social contingencies surrounding the research. Federal administrative law in place during the 1980s incorporated four key new provisions. First, it required subjects' consent for all experiments posing more than minimal risk. Distinctions between therapeutic and nontherapeutic intent and between patients and nonpatients no longer pertained.[7] Second, it specified that researchers were to fully inform subjects of the risks associated with experimental interventions and of available alternatives for medical treatments. Third, it imposed measures for ensuring that subjects' participation in research was voluntary. These included restrictions on experimentation with children, prisoners, and mental patients—groups whose capacities or circumstances might render them unable to consent freely. Fourth, federal regulations prohibited the inclusion in consent documents of clauses waiving subjects' legal rights—clauses common in consent forms used by the federal agencies funding wartime medical research.

The peer review established by DHHS codes also departed in significant ways from the professional and organizational practices that preceded it. Unlike the scientific panels used by research sponsors in the first half of the century, IRBs were located at institutions receiving research support rather than at organizations providing it. This had the effect of decoupling assessments of risk from decisions about funding. Furthermore, while many scientific advisory panels drew members from researchers working at a range of institutions who had expertise in a specialized area of medical science, IRBs drew their members from a small number of institutions—often only one—and a wide array of investigatory fields. Thus constituted, IRBs would often lack competency in the science underlying the protocols being reviewed.

When policy advocates recount the origins of federal regulation, they emphasize standards imposed from outside the research community. Changes in rules for consent did indeed originate outside prevailing scientific norms. Policymakers designed regulatory codes to bring consent practices in line with prevailing public sensibilities and with developments in the broader legal environment. These developments included the Nuremberg codes of 1947 and court rulings in malpractice cases issued during the late 1950s and early 1960s.[8] Meanwhile, shifts in the culture at large triggered the recalibration of parameters of justifiable hazards and a return to lesser-harm logic in the assessment of risks to subjects. Dangerous experiments without benefit for subjects were no longer acceptable.

But the medical-research community itself determined the structure of federal oversight and the location and character of IRBs. It was NIH policy that mandated local review boards in the 1960s. Although situated within a federal department, NIH has been constituted as a professional institution. Its directors, drawn from the elite of academic medicine, have both seen themselves and functioned as leaders of the medical-research community. In the early 1970s, NIH lobbied members of Congress to refrain from passing legislation that would fundamentally alter existing oversight structures. It sought to prevent the centralization of protocol review and the creation of a permanent bioethics commission. It succeeded not only in achieving these aims, but also in securing administrative purview over both local IRBs and the first national bioethics commission. For some time, these arrangements allowed the medical-research community to wield a large measure of control over the implementation of human-subjects regulations.[9]

From History to Theory

Throughout this book, I have underscored the fundamentally social nature of moral action by scientific communities. My central argument has been that researchers frame moral problems and impose—or decline to impose—moral constraints in the context of institutions and groups. I have examined patterns of oversight in two locales—the colleague network and the organization sponsoring clinical research—seldom explored as sites for moral decision making. My analysis reveals that a variety of social processes have powerfully affected how research networks and sponsors handle the of risk human research. Social dynamics have also given rise to new types of constraints and long-term change in the boundaries between acceptable and unacceptable experiments. In accounting for historical patterns in moral oversight, I have drawn on theoretical perspectives in the field of sociology. I now comment on the implications of my historical analysis for social-science theory.

Social Control within Professional and Scientific Communities

Sociologists have been in substantial disagreement about whether professions effectively control the conduct of their members. One line of thought points to dense informal rules bearing on the performance of work typical of professions whose members exercise high levels of autonomy. Practitioners' desire for the esteem of their colleagues, the argument goes, generates widespread conformity to group norms. This perspective follows Emile Durkheim's insight that occupational groups have distinctive moralities and engender solidarity.[10] Scholarship on professions dating from the mid-twentieth century emphasizes the collective identity and cohesion generated by occupational cultures. More recent contributors clarify norms operating within particular professions. Warren Hagstrom describes a well-embedded gift culture among scientists that governs patterns of exchange and peer recognition. Charles Bosk clarifies a tacit morality governing the performance of surgeons, norms grounded in work routines and relations between colleagues.[11]

A contrasting viewpoint emphasizes the shortcomings of informal controls and the lack of well-developed formal constraints. Eliot Freidson develops an extensive critique of regulation internal to medicine, pointing to both structural and normative impediments to the exercise of self-regulation by physicians. Freidson argues that the organization of medical practice makes it difficult for doctors to know how their colleagues are performing. Both the privacy of doctor-patient encounters and the nature of physician referral patterns impede the visibility of physicians' interactions with clients. Yet even where violations of professional standards are observable, he continues, doctors are loath to impose sanctions on colleagues. This is because physicians' cultural ethos emphasizes uncertainties in treating patients and the ever present possibility of medical error. As a result, doctors are reluctant to rebuke a colleague or take action to punish those who violate professional norms. Freidson also comments on limitations of the colleague boycott, which he identifies as the primary vehicle for informal control in medical practice. Here, doctors decline to refer their patients to a colleague who they judge to be substandard. Freidson underscores that this mechanism may protect the patients of the clinicians imposing the boycott, but it fails to protect patients more broadly.[12]

My account corroborates features of both major sociological perspectives on professional self-regulation, as they apply to scientific communities. I have suggested that research networks are a central locale for social control within science. These networks transcend work organizations and training centers—to date, the principal sites for studies of regulation within the professions. I have suggested that the character of scientific problem groups both encourages and undermines the exercise of informal controls. On the one hand, consistent with the findings of Hagstrom and Bosk, researchers' informal morality exerts a powerful influence on professional conduct. It generates frequent moral judgments and intense debate over the parameters of justifiable experimentation. Moral evaluations permeate scientific discourse on the safety and efficacy of medical interventions. My analysis adds two additional insights. First, medical researchers base their moral judgments on local knowledge: familiarity with the materials and techniques used in specialized arenas of science. Their assessments of the acceptability of risky human interventions rest on interpretations of empirical findings. Second, because of the technical character of disputes over local knowledge, the moral content of these debates is often not readily apparent to outside observers.

On the other hand, consistent with Freidson, there are serious shortcomings to self-regulation by medical researchers. I have pointed to several impediments to effective informal control that are not fully elaborated in the current literature. These include both uncertainties in interpreting scientific evidence and ambiguities that arise when norms are applied to particular situations. Authors addressing professional self-regulation typically assume that, if conduct is visible to peers, identifying deviance is unproblematic. But scientists often disagree about how to implement their moral standards. The loose-knit structure of colleague networks adds to difficulties in reaching consensuses about moral boundaries.

Moreover, even when scientists are in substantial agreement about what constitutes appropriate conduct, professional networks have limited tools for affecting members' behavior. While the disapproval of colleagues is a powerful deterrent for the great majority of researchers, problem groups have great difficulty constraining a member who, in the face of dissuasion, continues to insist on his or her own notion of acceptable conduct. When informal pressure fails to bring problematic research to a halt, there is little network members can do without assistance from outside. Ostracizing rule violators is an ineffective response. Scientists typically distance themselves from a colleague whose research they feel is overly hazardous. But informal pressures are most likely to influence scientists who are fully integrated into the research network, and least likely to affect those who are already marginal.

Research Institutions and Their Audiences

One of my key findings is that both scientists and their sponsors have undertaken sophisticated and sustained efforts to shape public culture bearing on human experimentation. For the research community, moral traditions have not only been standards for evaluating the appropriateness of risky interventions, but also rhetorical tools for justifying human research. Scientific leaders have invoked their traditions when endeavoring to discredit the claims of regulatory activists and to address public fears about hazardous medical procedures. They have presented laudatory accounts of human experimentation and sought to have these adopted in popular discourse.

Sociologists of science have pointed to other efforts by scientific leaders to influence the opinions of outside constituencies. Thomas Gieryn identifies a variety of ideological claims pursued episodically by researchers—what he calls "boundary-work"—involving the demarcation of science from non-science. Gieryn argues that scientists use boundary-work as a rhetorical strategy for enhancing the authority of science and the resources made available for its conduct.[13] The metaphor of boundaries has come into play in my discussion as well. I have argued that scientists generate rhetoric and imagery concerning moral boundaries in the conduct of human experiments. In my account, the most salient demarcations are not between science and non-science but, rather, between justifiable and unjustifiable research. Yet the two phenomena have more in common than a shared metaphor. In both boundary-work and the negotiation of moral boundaries, researchers seek to sustain the legitimacy and autonomy of science and to enhance resources for its conduct. In both, they orient their actions and direct their rhetoric toward affecting the views of important outside audiences.

That organizations try to influence their environment is also not a novel idea. Several scholars have shown that networks of organizations actively shape public policies for the institutional arena in which they participate. Others, examining the interface of organizations and the law, observe that when organizations adopt policies and procedures in response to ambiguous judicial or statutory mandates, these measures often become integrated into the letter of the law. Still others note that corporations routinely hire public relations consultants and undertake advertising campaigns.[14] What is remarkable about the efforts of research sponsors is how they went about shaping the environment. Their aim was no less than to define the terms of public discourse about human experiments. Following the lead of the professional community, sponsors of medical research generated a language and imagery depicting the methods of clinical research as appropriate and its goals as laudable. This rhetoric invoked highly valued cultural symbols. Organizational leaders sought to have these constructions prevail as dominant discourse in the popular media and other public arenas. Major research sponsors created special organizational units to coordinate efforts at persuasion.

I have suggested a number of reasons why medical-research communities and their sponsors have devoted resources to shaping popular sentiment. In the absence of public support, researchers might encounter difficulties sustaining resources, forestalling unwelcome regulation, and securing subjects. Moreover, members of the public have had an intense interest in the human use of medical innovations. They understand that medical experiments have immediate and tangible consequences for the health of subjects and long-term implications for the well-being of many others. Public fascination with experimental medical procedures is longstanding. In America, the news media have been providing extensive coverage of new clinical techniques since the 1880s.[15] But popular sentiments about medical innovation have been mercurial. Periodically, social movements and shifting ideological currents have undermined public trust. Research accidents have triggered widespread outcry. Meanwhile, perceptions of the acceptability of investigatory practices to outside audiences have been crucial to scientists' calculations about the assumption of risk. Clinical researchers and their sponsors share many of these vulnerabilities with the institutional communities that manage other hazardous products of science and technology. Not surprisingly, those communities also have devoted substantial resources to shaping public construction of and sentiments about risk.

Social Management of Risk

Controlling the risks of human experiments is one aspect of a larger social problem: how to handle the use of socially desirable but potentially hazardous technologies. A substantial body of literature has accumulated on societal responses to the dangers associated with applications of modern science. Scholars have examined the determinants of risk perceptions, the cultural constructions of danger, the social distribution of hazards, and social processes contributing to technological accidents. A core claim of sociological approaches to risk is that decision making about technological hazards is institutionally embedded, shaped by organizational dynamics and associated professional practices.[16] My analysis both builds on and contributes to this approach by clarifying patterns in the institutional management of hazards. More specifically, the preceding account suggests three additions to our understanding of the formal oversight of risk-laden technologies.

First, contemporaneous organizations can diverge markedly in their approaches to the same set of dangers. This happens where decision makers differ in the extent of their knowledgeability about risk and where organizations operate in distinctive market niches that generate divergent incentives and disincentives for undertaking hazardous activities. It happens also where organizations have had different experiences with public controversy. In these situations, organizations that are risk averse can coexist with those that are risk tolerant.

Second, the management of at least some technological hazards has evolved over time, becoming more organizationally embedded, more similar across organizations, and more highly formalized. These changes occur as the agencies that implement risky procedures and products respond to their professional, legal and organizational environments. Recent institutional theories provide tools for understanding such long-term developments in the management of hazardous technologies.

Third, when the state undertakes the regulation of technological hazards, it often draws from and relies heavily on existing institutional and professional norms. Sociologists have just begun to examine the relation between organizational rules and regulation imposed by the state through statutory and administrative law.[17] One implication of my analysis is that, in order to understand how government regulation evolves, scholars also need to understand fully the origins and character of informal and institutionally embedded controls that precede and coexist with official oversight. This argument is compatible with recent empirical research on the emergence of consumer safety regulations. In that regulatory arena as well, informal and institutionally embedded controls have arisen before political advocacy for governmental controls. Furthermore, federal regulatory code has incorporated institutional rules and delegated regulatory functions to institutional bodies.[18]

Moral Traditions in Historical Perspective

My observations about change over time in research oversight raise questions about the continuing status of moral traditions among medical scientists. Has the advent of government regulation undermined the community's observance of its informal morality? Or have developments internal to medical science—in the culture, methods, or organization of research networks—altered the content of researchers' traditions or the character of their expression? Available evidence bearing on these questions, particularly the first one, is sparse. But several trends are accessible to observation.

One such trend is a decline in the importance of self-experimentation. Lawrence Altman cites instances of the practice through the middle decades of the twentieth century.[19] But examples from the final third of the century are harder to find. An NIH policy issued in 1953 prohibited self-experimentation by in-house researchers.[20] I have suggested that self-experimentation had its origins in nineteenth-century notions linking professionalism to personal honor and character. But by the 1950s, for an investigator to serve also as human subject was out of step with the medical-research communities' growing commitment to scientific criteria and acceptance of randomized clinical trials. Moreover, public confidence in the products of medical science was sufficiently high after midcentury that demonstrations of researchers' personal honor may have no longer seemed necessary.

Another long-term trend concerns patterns of moral stewardship. Early-twentieth-century medical leaders were quite willing to exert pressure on colleagues about matters related to investigatory conduct. Simon Flexner, scientific director of the prestigious Rockefeller Institution for Medical Research from 1906 through 1935, acted as moral arbiter within the polio-research community. Flexner initiated a moratorium on human testing of polio vaccines and, for more than two decades, took personal responsibility for seeing that medical scientists observed it. He wrote numerous letters to contemporary researchers warning against clinical use of poliovirus or other investigatory practices that might result in human injury. When he felt that his message had not gotten across, Flexner would intervene through an investigator's colleague or mentor. I find little evidence of this type of professional stewardship among researchers during final third of the century.

But if scientists became more reluctant in the second half of the twentieth century to engage in private intrusions into the professional affairs of colleagues, they also became more willing to engage in public moral debate and to criticize colleagues in arenas visible to outsiders. Through the early 1940s, professional leaders endeavored to suppress information about human experimentation that might fuel critics with regulatory agendas. This included keeping intraprofessional disputes over research conduct out of public view.[21] In contrast, during the 1960s and 1970s, researchers were engaging in open disputes over investigatory conduct. Some of these took place in the editorial pages of major medical journals.[22] Others spilled out into public arenas. These conflicts—and the erosion of agreements among clinical researchers about the rules for conducting human experiments—were the principal reason that NIH initiated federal research oversight and supported the codification of new guidelines for the conduct of human experiments.

In the final third of the twentieth century, debate within public arenas became increasingly important to decisions about human applications of experimental procedures. Renée Fox and Judith Swazey note that, when compared with clinical moratoria occurring before 1980, later suspensions depended more on pressures from bioethicists and lay audiences, exerted in good measure through the mass media.[23] A number of developments have contributed to the heightened salience of public arenas to decisions about the conduct of human experiments. These include the advent of bioethics and regulatory law; pressures from newly mobilized constituencies of patients; continued growth in the importance of federal funding to the conduct of medical research; and expansion in NIH's role in formulating clinical-research policy.[24] As these trends have unfolded, the social processes shaping the construction of public problems have become even more significant in the framing and resolution of moral issues in the conduct of human experiments.[25] Lesser-harm logic and its correlates have been viable and fully operative since the late nineteenth century. But today, informal processes within communities of medical scientists are only one among many dynamics affecting the conduct of human experiments.

Moral Traditions in an Era of Government Oversight

What relevance do professional traditions and organizational practices of the early and middle decades of the twentieth century have for current research-oversight policies? Today's human-subjects researchers conform to regulatory codes administered by two federal agencies: the Food and Drug Administration (FDA) and the Office for Human Research Protections (OHRP). The FDA oversees human testing of experimental drugs, biological materials, and medical devices. It has done so since the early 1960s, when Congress mandated that the FDA not only license medical products, but also control the use of those undergoing clinical testing. FDA codes require that the sponsor of an experimental product obtain an exemption from federal licensing laws—called an investigational new drug (IND) exemption—before conducting human experiments. Agency procedures structure clinical testing into three phases, with review of sponsor-provided data on safety and efficacy intervening between stages. Meanwhile, researchers must report adverse events among subjects that occur during human trials.

The OHRP oversees a system of institutional review boards (IRBs), committees that scrutinize human-subjects studies to be conducted at universities, hospitals, and other institutions that receive federal research support. IRBs date to the late 1960s, when the National Institutes of Health (NIH) initiated local review of human-subjects research supported by NIH funds. In 1974, NIH's parent agency, then the U.S. Department of Health, Education, and Welfare, issued federal regulatory codes mandating IRB review of human-subjects research conducted under its aegis. These codes prescribed the composition and operation of the IRBs and detailed criteria to be used for evaluating research protocols. That year, Congress also passed legislation creating the National Commission for the Protection of Human Subjects of Biomedical and Behavioral Research and charged it with further elaborating IRB codes. Members of the emerging field of bioethics played a central role in formulating principles for research oversight through their appointments on the National Commission and on subsequent federally mandated bioethics panels. Resulting federal administrative law has directed IRBs to pay particular attention to researchers' plans for selecting and recruiting subjects, procedures for securing the informed consent of subjects, and the balance of risks and benefits of proposed experiments.

Now that officially mandated regulation is in place, have not the procedures implemented by the FDA and OHRP superseded the professional and organizational practices of the early twentieth century? And have not the principles articulated by national bioethics commissions supplanted the research community's informal morality? If so, what does it matter how scientists and research sponsors more than a half-century ago handled research oversight and the moral problems attending human experimentation?

I argue that scientists' moral traditions have immediate relevance for current regulatory policy. Researchers' traditions are not merely relics of the past. They continue to operate today, albeit in modified forms, alongside both state-mandated oversight and principles advanced by the bioethics community. As detailed earlier in this book, scientists' informal morality insists that experiments be technically sound, that animal testing precede human trials, and that the hazards of a medical intervention be lower than the risk of the natural disease. The strengths of scientists' informal oversight include the competency of problem-group members to evaluate investigatory hazards, their readiness to exchange views about the implications of empirical findings, and their sense of collective responsibility—not always readily marshaled—for avoiding serious research injuries. I maintain that for government regulation to be optimally effective, it must build on core features and strengths of scientists' informal morality. Where formal oversight stints or obstructs scientists' longstanding traditions, it is likely to generate regulatory failures.

I develop this line of argument by examining two recent clinical experiments that resulted in research-induced fatalities. The scientific bases of these experiments lie far afield from that underlying the vaccine trials of the early and mid-twentieth century. But the issues these contemporary experiments raise are entirely compatible with my focus on human risk and research oversight.

Accounting for Research Fatalities

Events surrounding the deaths of two research subjects, one at the University of Pennsylvania in 1999 and another at Johns Hopkins University in 2001, point to fundamental limitations of state-mandated oversight of medical research. In the first of these cases, the subject, eighteen-year-old Jesse Gelsinger, was a participant in the trial of a gene-transfer intervention for treatment of ornithine transcarbamylase (OTC) deficiency, a genetic disorder in which the liver fails to produce an enzyme necessary for the breakdown of ammonia, a byproduct of metabolism. High blood-ammonia levels associated with OTC deficiency can cause coma, brain damage, and death. Many of those born with a severe form of the disease die early in infancy. The genetic intervention being tested by Penn researchers was aimed at stimulating temporary production of the missing enzyme by infusing the livers of affected patients with corrective genetic material. Gelsinger died from an acute inflammatory reaction to the study's adenovirus vector—the preparation used to deliver the corrective genes. At the time, he was in no danger of succumbing to his genetic disorder. Gelsinger had partial OTC deficiency. His condition was stable, controlled by drugs and a low-protein diet.

In the second case, Ellen Roche, age twenty-four, was a subject in an experiment examining the physiology of asthma conducted at the Johns Hopkins Bayview Medical Center. When people without asthma inhale deeply, their bronchial muscles relax, causing their airways to dilate. This response protects against the airway constriction and hyperreactivity that characterize asthmatic episodes. Hopkins researchers hypothesized that bronchial-wall nerves control airway dilation, and that the functioning of these nerves is defective in asthmatics. Investigators sought to confirm this model by demonstrating that, in healthy subjects, blockage of bronchial-nerve ganglia would suppress the airway dilation that typically accompanies deep inhalation. Their experiment involved administering the nerve-blocking agent hexamethonium into the respiratory tracts of healthy subjects. In Roche, the agent's impact went well beyond temporary disruption of bronchial-wall ganglia. It resulted in lung damage, respiratory distress syndrome, and ultimately, multiple organ failure and death.

Gelsinger and Roche died as a consequence of experimental procedures. Both were healthy or medically stable before their participation. Neither had much to gain from the interventions they were receiving. The Hopkins study had no therapeutic intent. In the case of the Penn experiment, even if the gene therapy stimulated temporary OTC production—critics say it did not— researchers knew it was unlikely that the procedure could be used effectively on the same patient a second time. A characteristic of the vector Penn researchers were using was that the body's immune system inactivates it upon multiple exposures. If benefits to subjects in these experiments were minimal, the risks were grave. Comments from members of the scientific community after the accidents make it clear that the researchers initiating the two experiments had greatly underestimated investigatory hazards.

It is striking that these experiments proceeded, despite their inauspicious balance of risks and benefits, when the formal regulatory system was fully in place. Both groups of researchers had submitted their protocols to their university IRBs and had received clearances to proceed. The Penn investigators had obtained the required exemption from the FDA. They had also undergone scrutiny by the NIH's Recombinant DNA Advisory Committee (RAC)—established in 1974. Consistent with NIH policy, between the late 1980s and mid-1990s, the RAC conducted case-by-case review of all NIH supported gene-therapy trials. How regulatory bodies came to approve the two experiments—risks and benefit ratios notwithstanding—reveals much about our current oversight system and prevailing evaluative standards, as do the responses of regulatory agencies to the experiments' unfortunate outcomes.

The University of Pennsylvania Experiment

Three physician-investigators collaborated on the University of Pennsylvania OTC trial: Mark Batshaw, a pediatrician with considerable experience treating OTC deficiency; Steven Raper, a surgeon who administered the experiment's gene-transfer preparation; and James M. Wilson, the bench scientist who developed and oversaw laboratory testing of the study's adenovirus vector. Wilson was a highly respected figure in the gene-therapy research community. He directed the University of Pennsylvania Institute for Human Gene Therapy (IHGT), sponsor of the Penn OTC trial and one of the largest gene-therapy laboratories in the country. In 1999, the IHGT had a budget of $25 million.[1]

Wilson and Batshaw began work on a gene-transfer intervention for OTC deficiency when Wilson arrived at Penn in 1993. The field of gene therapy was still in its early years. It was in 1990 that a team headed by W. French Anderson conducted the first federally approved human intervention with a genetically engineered preparation. The first human use of an adenovirus vector—for treatment of cystic fibrosis—took place 1992. Adenovirus vectors were one of several types of gene-transfer preparations that researchers were developing in the 1990s. At the end of that decade, the FDA had, under its purview, 204 active INDs for gene-therapy products. Of these, about 30 percent involved adenovirus vectors.[2]

The Penn study was a phase I clinical trial—an experiment to test safety and determine appropriate dosage levels for future trials. It was the first to deliver an adenovirus vector to asymptomatic or stable patients. Wilson's goal was to determine the "maximum tolerated dose" of the vector, high enough to optimize OTC expression but low enough to avoid serious side effects. The study design involved administering increasing amounts of the vector to six successive cohorts of subjects. Penn investigators received RAC approval to proceed with their experiment in December of 1995. They treated their first subject in April of 1997. Gelsinger's intervention took place in September of 1999. He was the eighteenth subject, the second in the study's final cohort. Gelsinger and the previous participant received vector dosages three hundred times higher than the first group of subjects—the highest doses of adenovirus vector ever used with human recipients. Researchers performed Gelsinger's gene transfer on September 13. They removed his life-support equipment four days later, on September 17.

After Gelsinger's death, the FDA placed an immediate halt on the OTC experiment, and both it and the RAC began investigations. In subsequent months, the FDA issued warning letters and initiated corrective action, Congress held hearings on gene-therapy oversight, Penn conducted an internal review and reached an out-of-court settlement with Gelsinger's family, and members of the gene-therapy research community engaged in public soul searching. These events generated widespread media coverage.

The FDA took the lead in issuing regulatory findings. It charged the Penn researchers with multiple violations. They had failed to report that several subjects treated before Gelsinger, with lower doses of the vector, showed signs of stage-three liver damage following the intervention. Proceeding with additional subjects after such reactions violated the experiment's stopping rules. And reporting serious adverse events during clinical testing was an FDA requirement. There were other infractions as well. Researchers had made changes in the experimental protocol, relaxing patient-inclusion requirements, without FDA approval. They had neglected to perform pretrial and follow-up tests on subjects, as specified in the protocol. They did not provide the agency with timely information about the deaths of monkeys in experiments with a closely related adenovirus vector. They had failed to fully inform research subjects of experimental hazards, withholding information about both animal deaths and adverse events among earlier patients.[3]

The federal response to Gelsinger's death was not limited to initiating action against Penn researchers. Regulatory agencies took measures to ensure the safety of other gene-therapy experiments. The FDA placed holds not only on the Penn OTC experiment, but also on several other adenoviral-vector trials. It undertook a study of regulatory compliance among gene-therapy researchers. Both the FDA and the RAC moved to enforce adverse-event reporting requirements. Both undertook scientific reassessments of the safety of adenovirus vectors. But a principal thrust of the federal response was to identify procedural violations on the part of researchers and pursue disciplinary action. In May of 2000, the University of Pennsylvania announced corrective measures: neither Wilson nor the IHGT would conduct further clinical trials; their activities would be restricted to basic-science research.

The Johns Hopkins Experiment

Alkis Togias, associate professor of clinical immunology, directed the Johns Hopkins asthma study. The experiment took place at the university's Asthma and Allergy Center under a grant from the NIH Heart, Lung, and Blood Institute. The grant's principal investigator was Solbert Permutt, a pulmonary specialist whose earlier work provided the basis for the study's model of bronchial dilation. Togias was coinvestigator on the grant and lead researcher of the hexamethonium experiment. It was he who enrolled Ellen Roche—at the time, employed as a technician at the Asthma Center.

Togias's protocol called for administering by inhalation one gram of hexamethonium to a small number of healthy subjects. He chose hexamethonium as a nerve-blocking agent because it was known to suppress the type of ganglia that he and Permutt believed to be operative in bronchial dilation. Physicians once used hexamethonium intravenously during surgery as a means for controlling high blood pressure and bleeding. But other medications superseded its application for these purposes, and in 1972, the FDA classified it as an unapproved substance. Togias stated later that he had made inquiries into whether FDA approval would be necessary for his use of hexamethonium. He was not testing the substance as a therapeutic agent and, in the end, did not seek an IND exemption—this would be a point of contention with the FDA. The Hopkins IRB approved Togias's research protocol in September 2000. He administered hexamethonium to his first subject in April 2001. Roche was the third subject in the study. She received the experimental intervention on May 4, 2001. In the days that followed, Roche developed progressively more serious symptoms. On May 9, she was hospitalized at Bayview Medical Center, where she died on June 2.

Roche's death triggered inquiries by internal and external review committees at Johns Hopkins, and investigations by the FDA and the OHRP. FDA staff faulted Togias for not securing an IND exemption, but the agency delayed official action against the researcher. It was the OHRP that issued the government's principal regulatory findings, and it targeted the conduct of both Togias and the Hopkins IRB. In the letter dated July 19, 2001, the OHRP faulted Togias for missing crucial findings on the risks of hexamethonium. When reviewing literature on the substance's use, Togias had failed to cite published studies indicating that hexamethonium, when inhaled, could cause lung damage, even though this information was "readily available via routine ... data searches, as well as recent textbooks on the pathology of the lung."[4] The OHRP pointed to other lapses as well. Togias had not assured that the hexamethonium given to subjects was sufficiently pure for human use. He had failed to submit an adverse-event report to the Hopkins IRB when, after the experimental intervention, the study's first subject developed a cough—Togias attributed the subject's symptoms to the flu. Before Roche's intervention, Togias had altered his method of administering hexamethonium—accelerating the rate of delivery—without first seeking approval from the Hopkins IRB. And the study's consent form was inadequate. The document failed to state that hexamethonium was an unapproved drug, that its use as an inhalant was experimental, or that the substance, when inhaled, might pose a danger of lung damage.

OHRP officials determined that the Hopkins IRB shared responsibility for several of these infractions. The board was remiss in failing to identify research findings linking hexamethonium to lung damage. It should have required assurance of the chemical's purity for clinical use and insisted on a fuller account of experimental hazards in the study's consent document. Furthermore, regulators found that the operating procedures of the Hopkins IRB were seriously flawed. Subcommittees were handling initial protocol review, without discussion at convened meetings of the board as a whole. And the board had failed to keep minutes of deliberations about individual research protocols. On July 19, 2001, the OHRP temporarily suspended human-subjects research at Johns Hopkins School of Medicine until the institution submitted a plan for corrective action. In this plan, the School of Medicine agreed to overhaul the operating procedures of its IRB and to reevaluate twenty-six hundred human-subjects protocols.[5]

An Alternative Perspective

Regulatory agencies investigating the deaths of Gelsinger and Roche looked for and found procedural violations. They faulted researchers at Penn and

Hopkins, as well as the Hopkins IRB, for failures of compliance. Their official findings did not address larger issues about the adequacy of the oversight system itself. But the two experiments do raise several fundamental questions about government oversight of clinical research. Does the federal regulatory system adequately bring to bear available knowledge for assessing investigatory risks? And do prevailing evaluative standards provide an appropriate balance of research benefits and hazards? My analysis points to four persistent problems that either are left unresolved by the current oversight system or are endemic to it. These problems may have contributed to the research fatalities at Penn and Hopkins.

The Need for Expert Assessment of Risk

The first problem is that, for a large portion of medical experiments, official oversight fails to mobilize expert assessments of research hazards. This is very often the case for experiments evaluated only by IRBs. Federal codes direct local review boards to consider the balance of risks and benefits when making decisions about protocol approval. Members of these committees are ostensibly peers of the scientists who initiate research protocols. In some ways then, IRB review is similar to the informal assessments of risks undertaken by investigatory communities. But the oversight of local review boards differs in consequential ways from that exercised by scientific problem groups. Researchers' moral traditions place the burden of risk assessment with the geographically dispersed network of scientists who share experience with the materials and techniques used in developing and testing a medical intervention. These scientists have the knowledge and skills to make evaluations of hazards independent of those offered by the investigators who initiate a human experiment. In contrast, IRBs draw their scientific members from a very small number of institutions and a very broad range of research fields. Thus constituted, these boards lack the expertise to make technically competent estimates for the risks of the great bulk of protocols that fall within their purview. Where no board member is an expert in the science underlying an experiment, and where the study's investigators are well-regarded medical researchers, IRBs are likely to defer to the risk assessments offered by the protocol's authors.

It is an unfortunate fact about the events preceding Roche's death that information linking hexamethonium and lung damage was readily available in published sources and was common knowledge among at least a portion of respiratory researchers, and yet neither the study's principal investigator nor the Hopkins IRB was aware of this evidence. But faulting the Hopkins

IRB for failing to recognize the chemical's toxicity is to overlook how such boards are composed. IRBs are not designed to bring to bear available knowledge about investigatory hazards. Moreover, when venturing their own assessments of risk, IRBs are likely to misperceive hazards, and not always in the direction of underestimating severity.[6]

I have underscored throughout this book that colleague networks have serious limitations as a vehicle for research oversight. Scientists often disagree in their interpretations of empirical findings pertaining to investigatory hazards. They may be reluctant to criticize a problem-group member lest their statements appear motivated by professional jealousy or they are proven wrong by later research. Not all scientists are fully integrated into colleague networks, and not all networks are equally equipped to effect social control. Even when a problem group moves to restrain a member's conduct, the pressures it exerts are informal ones.

All this being said, the historical record shows that it is possible to design oversight structures that deploy the strengths of the colleague network and avoid some of its shortcomings. During the middle decades of the twentieth century, organizations sponsoring medical research created scientific advisory panels that quite effectively monitored the hazards of clinical trials. Scientific panels like those at the National Foundation for Infantile Paralysis included experts in the relevant fields of medical research. These committees coupled decisions about scientific quality, the inauguration of human testing, and project support. They drew on researchers' informal traditions, adding a straightforward means—control over funding—for delaying or stopping clinical experiments judged to be too hazardous. At their best, scientific advisory boards mobilized the research community's specialized competencies for evaluating risk, and its sense of collective responsibility for avoiding human injury.

Federally mandated oversight of clinical research will do an optimal job of preventing human injury only when it assigns judgments about research risks to scientists competent to make such assessments. One way to effectively organize such review is through the use of centralized advisory panels composed of experts in the specialized fields underlying the protocols being reviewed. Such panels might serve another function as well. Critics of the IRB system note that, by placing decisions about protocol approval with local review boards, it provides no general forum for addressing the wisdom of proceeding with human use of untested medical interventions.[7] Centralized scientific review boards might play a role in generating publicly accessible commentary on both the promise and liabilities of newly emerging medical technologies.

Complexities in Managing Scientific Review

A second set of problems concerns the design and management of specialized scientific review of human-subjects protocols. While IRBs lack the expertise to evaluate research hazards, the same cannot be said of the NIH's RAC or the FDA. Both agencies reviewed the Penn OTC protocol, and both had access to specialists in the field of gene therapy. But even where regulatory arrangements provide for expert assessment of risk, the design and management of this input has been problematic. Policymakers designed the RAC to address ethical issues surrounding the application of new genetic technologies—creating a national forum absent for most arenas of medical science. RAC members include scientific specialists, bioethicists, and individuals chosen to voice concerns of the public—most of whom represent patient advocacy groups. In the mid-1980s, the RAC set up procedures for case-by-case review of gene-therapy protocols—at first through its Human Gene Therapy Subcommittee and then, beginning in 1992, through the committee as a whole.[8] Meanwhile, the FDA remains the principal agency regulating experimental use of medical products. It requires that clinical researchers secure an IND exemption before undertaking the human testing of new genetically engineered preparations. The agency's in-house scientific staff evaluates IND protocols and accompanying evidence on safety and efficacy provided by the applicant. The FDA also has standing scientific advisory panels that it can consult in the course of making decisions about protocol approval.

Approval by the RAC and FDA notwithstanding, after Gelsinger's death, commentators questioned whether the study's researchers and reviewers had fully considered available information on the hazards of adenovirus vectors. Deborah Nelson and Rick Weiss, staff writers for the *Washington Post*, interviewed members of the gene-therapy research community, who pointed to troubling data about the vectors' safety. Some of this came to light following the protocol's formal approval. Nelson and Weiss write:

> Between the start of the [Penn] clinical trial and Gelsinger's death . . . new research elsewhere in the field provided further evidence of toxicity and the need for caution in using adenovirus in the liver. "Not many people consider it appropriate for treating genetic disease," said NIH investigator Richard Morrow. The NIH tested a closely related adenovirus on the livers of three macaque monkeys, which fell seriously ill with symptoms similar to those that killed Gelsinger. They recovered, but one suffered permanent liver damage. A German study involving similar adenoviruses caused

acute, toxic responses in rabbits that also, resembled those that killed Gelsinger. [Guenter] Cichon, the Berlin researcher who led the study, concluded that adenoviruses should be used only in dire circumstances. . . . To give adenoviruses to patients like Gelsinger "would never be justified," Cichon said. "And I am not the only one who thinks this way. We do not understand why [researchers] are taking these risks."[9]

There were other critics from within the scientific community. Richard Mulligan, a Harvard University molecular biologist who developed new gene-splicing techniques in the late 1970s, faulted Wilson for stinting on his animal research. Mulligan reviewed Wilson's data for the RAC, after the Penn experiment was shut down. He discovered that Wilson had failed to examine exactly how and why extremely high doses of his adenovirus vector caused death in monkeys. Wilson was satisfied simply to use lower doses in humans.[10] Other researchers pointed to longstanding evidence that adenovirus vectors could cause severe inflammation. Some wondered whether they should have spoken out before Gelsinger's death against human use of very high doses of such vectors.[11]

Clearly, these commentators had the benefit of hindsight. It is a great deal easier to identify overlooked signs of hazards in the aftermath of a human injury than it is to evaluate the implications of such signs before an accident's occurrence. The fact that human harm occurs does not necessarily mean that prior assessments of risks and benefits were mishandled. Still, such observations by members of the research community cast doubt on the wisdom of approving the Penn OTC protocol. Were the RAC and FDA fully aware of the scientific community's concerns about the vector's safety? Was the review process structured to discover these concerns and bring them to bear in decisions about protocol approval?

Records of the RAC show that its review did raise relevant questions about the risks of adenovirus vectors. Consistent with the committee's procedures, three members served as primary reviewers, preparing comments on the Penn OTC protocol for presentation to the RAC as a whole. One of these reviewers, Robert Erickson, professor of pediatrics and molecular biology at the University of Arizona Medical School, emphasized the possibility for a severe inflammation, particularly when the vector was delivered directly to the liver. He also noted the ineffectiveness of the vector in generating long-term OTC expression. Rochelle Hirschhorn, professor of medicine and cell biology at New York University and another RAC reviewer, pointed to both the possibility of inflammatory reactions and the unlikelihood that the vector could be used safely or effectively for repeated applications. But the RAC was persuaded by Wilson's presentation at their December 1995 meeting. Wilson was very highly regarded within the scientific community. He argued that his newly developed vectors solved problems associated with earlier generations of adenovirus preparations. And he promised revisions to the protocol—later reversed by the FDA—whereby the vector would be delivered through an intravenous line rather than into subjects' hepatic artery.[12]

While documents show that the RAC's evaluation identified hazards entailed in the Penn OTC experiment, they also reveal that the committee's purview was circumscribed. In assessing research protocols, the RAC's mandate was to address ethical issues and the balance of risks and benefits in the conduct of human gene-therapy trials. It was not set up to conduct full-scale scientific reviews as do NIH study groups. Nor was it equipped to require toxicity or other laboratory tests prior to human trials, or to provide hands-on oversight of ongoing clinical research. Before Gelsinger's death, the RAC addressed the Penn OTC protocol only once. At the time, Wilson had not yet finished developing the third generation of adenovirus vector that his research team eventually used with patients.[13] RAC approval of the Penn protocol (in December 1995) took place more than a year before the researchers ran their first human subject (in April 1997), and nearly four years before Gelsinger's treatment (in September 1999).

The RAC's mandate did include collecting reports on adverse events from ongoing gene-therapy trials and making these available to the research community. But in the months following approval of the Penn OTC protocol, the NIH Office of Recombinant DNA Activities was not enforcing RAC reporting requirements, and its data-collection functions were largely inoperative. At the time, the NIH was reevaluating the RAC's mandate with the aim of scaling back its role in protocol approval. Pressures from at least three directions lay behind this initiative. First, the National Task Force on AIDS Drug Development objected to dual RAC/FDA review as an obstacle to the timely development of new treatments for AIDS. Second, gene-therapy researchers complained that review of protocols by both the RAC and the FDA was duplicative and unnecessarily burdensome. Third, the leadership of the NIH had its own reasons for wanting to curtail the RAC's role in protocol review. Many of the investigators spearheading gene-therapy studies—Wilson among them—received at least some of their funding from biotechnology firms. Harold Varmus, then NIH head, did not wish to lend the NIH's imprimatur to industry research. Varmus felt that much of the science underlying gene-therapy trials was insufficiently strong to justify human trials, and that RAC approval of protocols was serving to legitimize clinical testing.[14]

In 1997, the NIH stripped the RAC of its protocol-approval authority and reconstituted it as an advisory body that would conduct case-by-case review of only controversial gene-therapy studies. Officially, the RAC retained its role in collecting and posting adverse-event reports from ongoing experiments. In fact, the NIH office that supported the RAC's work was not performing these functions. In the aftermath of Gelsinger's death, the NIH announced its intention of enforcing RAC reporting requirements, and it received hundreds of adverse-event reports in a matter of weeks. At the time of Gelsinger's intervention, the RAC had no apparatus in place for gathering and disseminating information bearing on the risks of vectors undergoing testing. Nor was there a mechanism for reevaluating ongoing protocols in light of new findings bearing on safety.

Review by the FDA has also had limitations. This agency assigns oversight of gene-therapy protocols to its Center for Biologics Evaluation and Research (CBER), which, like the FDA more broadly, employs a staff-scientist system rather than an advisory-committee model for reviewing experimental protocols. The CBER does have a scientific panel with expertise in gene-transfer research. For some years, its Biological Response Modifiers Advisory Committee (BRMAC) has included one or more gene-therapy specialists on its roster. But the BRMAC's purview extends well beyond this area. The committee also addresses—and includes experts on—organ transplantation and transmission of animal viruses. Furthermore, while the CBER calls on its advisory panels to assist in licensing decisions and in developing guidelines for the evaluation of categories of IND applications, it seldom consults with a panel about authorization of individual clinical trials.

Instead, in-house scientists handle the case-by-case review of phase I gene-therapy protocols. During the late 1980s and early 1990s, the CBER expanded its professional staff in fields bearing on the evaluation of genetically engineered products. It created the Division of Cellular and Gene Therapy (DCGT) in 1992. DCGT staff scientists—Ph.D.'s and M.D.'s— serve either as full-time regulators or as researcher-reviewers who pursue their own research agendas, much like university-based investigators, while devoting a portion of their time to regulatory activities. A combination of active researchers and desk scientists evaluate protocols for phase-one gene-therapy trials.[15] A team of three examines each application for an IND exemption. Teams include a product reviewer (addressing issues in manufacture of genetic products), a pharmacology-toxicology reviewer (examining data from animal and other laboratory studies), and a clinical reviewer (focusing on procedures to be followed in the course of human testing). When the DCGT grants an exemption for a phase I trial, it often does so with the stipulation that investigators observe protocol-specific rules for dose escalation and stopping. Researchers are to follow these rules and report adverse events that arise during testing.

A potential shortcoming of the FDA's staff-scientist model of oversight relates to the fit between protocols and competencies of reviewers. While the DCGT receives a large volume of protocols for a broad range of products, the CBER's budget places limits on the number of DCGT staff scientists. Inevitably, staff reviewers have more knowledge of some fields than others, and they are sometimes evaluating protocols outside their core competencies. When this happens, the staff members responsible for protocol evaluation are likely to be considerably less informed about issues bearing on safety than are scientists actively engaged in related arenas of research. The DCGT handles this in part by building checks into its authorizations—like the product-specific rules for dose escalation and stopping.

The most serious limitation of FDA oversight is that the agency treats virtually all information about IND protocols as proprietary, to be revealed only by a product's sponsor. The FDA has a dual statutory mandate: to protect public safety and to allow for the expeditious introduction of new commercial products. Political pressures shape how FDA officials reconcile these often conflicting imperatives, and the results often favor the corporate interests of product sponsors. The handling of information about clinical testing of experimental products is an area where corporate interests have prevailed. The FDA publishes the warning letters it has issued to investigators and sponsors it has found to be in violation of regulatory codes. But its nondisclosure policy on IND protocols extends to research findings bearing on product safety—including reports of adverse events from clinical trials—except where there is compelling public interest for disclosure. DCGT staff often work with the RAC to make some information about gene-therapy trials publicly available, since RAC review, unlike FDA oversight, is open to outside scrutiny. But even in the case of the Penn OTC trial, where the FDA made public disclosures concerning safety, the great bulk of records on FDA review and authorization remain inaccessible.[16] This policy makes it impossible for an observer outside the agency to evaluate in any depth whether the FDA's oversight of a particular protocol was flawed.

Managing the oversight of research hazards by technically competent scientists involves numerous complexities. Is the staff-scientist or advisory-panel model a preferable design? If staff scientists are to be used, how close should the expertise of evaluators be to the science underlying proposed clinical trials? If advisory panels are employed, how are the appropriate parameters of research fields to be determined? On what basis should scientists be chosen to serve on panels, and who should be charged with doing the selecting? How much and what type of oversight should take place after protocol approval, during the conduct of a clinical trial? Under what circumstances should information about adverse events from new human or animal trials lead to a halt in already approved IND research? Who should make such determinations? How best to handle these issues is by no means obvious.[17]

An undoubted shortcoming of the current system is, however, apparent. The policies of the FDA—policies consistent with its statutory mandate—actively obstruct the dissemination of findings bearing on investigatory hazards. A serious consequence is that members of the broader research community are denied information relevant to their assessment of the risks of ongoing and prospective human experiments. Regulation will be fully effective at preventing human injury only when it provides the scientific community with unimpeded access to evidence on adverse events during human testing and on the outcome of clinical trials.

Losing Sight of Lesser Harms

A third problem is that the evaluative standards used by regulatory bodies have stinted the importance of lesser-harm logic. A striking feature of the Penn experiment was the researchers' deliberate choice to draw subjects from among adults who were stable or asymptomatic, with partial OTC deficiency, rather than infants with life-threatening forms of the disease. In doing so, the scientists were stepping outside the longstanding tradition whereby the risks of an experimental intervention must be lower then the risks of the natural disease. According to this logic, it might be acceptable to give terminally ill patients a hazardous preparation, one with only a small chance of conferring benefit, but administering the same preparation to asymptomatic subjects would be unjustifiable.

When the RAC evaluated the Penn OTC protocol, the study's subject pool was a point of contention. The two RAC reviewers who voiced concern about the risks of Wilson's vector also raised questions about the appropriateness of experimenting on asymptomatic subjects. Rochelle Hirschhorn objected to the use of patients "not in a class . . . where fatal or neurological impaired outcomes were virtually inevitable."[18] Robert Erickson observed that "the treatment is potentially toxic" and yet it "is to be given to a target population who are nearly asymptomatic." According to RAC minutes, "Erickson found that the proposal using this asymptomatic patient population is not justified." He "would consider it to be more acceptable if . . . the treatment is given to affected children with life threatening OTC deficiency."[19]

Why, then, did the Penn research team choose, and the RAC approve, use of subjects with asymptomatic OTC deficiency? The Penn team presented two rationales for selecting this subject pool. One was that an experiment with adults would yield more useful scientific information. Children with total OTC deficiency would be acutely ill and the conditions surrounding their treatment would be very difficult to control. Batshaw and Wilson maintained that "the chance of obtaining valid scientific data is much greater in a planned study than in an unplanned emergency situation where an infant may arrive in a coma and from another institution."[20]

But it was a different argument that persuaded the RAC. The Penn researchers insisted that it was preferable to use adult subjects for ethical and humanitarian reasons. A bioethics consultant had advised them that it would be difficult for the parents of infants with fatal OTC deficiency to make an uncoerced decision about having their child participate in a research study. As Batshaw and Wilson explained:

> Our choice represents that endorsed by the bioethicists. . . . Informed consent can better be obtained from a clinically stable adult than from a parent whose infant is in the midst of a life-threatening crisis. We do not deny a potential for the appearance of coercion in an asymptomatic . . . adult, however, this potential is substantially diminished when compared to the couple with an acutely ill infant.[21]

The researchers also noted that an advocacy group composed of parents of OTC children endorsed the selection of adult subjects.[22] At the RAC meeting that approved the Penn protocol, members chosen to represent the public argued that, to show sympathy for the young victims of OTC deficiency, adult patients should assume risks for the children. For patient advocacy groups and some bioethicists, sympathy for the youngest victims and concerns with informed consent took priority over lesser harms. And securing input from these constituencies was a central reason for the RAC's existence.

Giving informed consent primacy over lesser harms departs sharply from the longstanding priorities of the medical-research community. Scientists' moral traditions have placed much greater emphasis on the control of research hazards than on the consent of subjects. Early-twentieth-century medical leaders recognized the importance of consent in American law, and they urged clinical investigators to secure the consent of subjects in medical research. Some of the organizations sponsoring mid-twentieth-century clinical trials required that investigators use written consent statements. But these statements often failed to protect human subjects. Researchers routinely drew subjects from custodial institutions without questioning whether participation of inmates was genuinely voluntary. And consent documents typically included waiver provisions that released researchers and sponsors from liability for human injury.

Regulatory and legal change during the second half of the twentieth century largely reversed these priorities. Federal regulatory codes prohibited use of waiver provisions in consent documents and created protections for institutionalized and other vulnerable subjects. In the courts, informed consent became the answer to medical hazards. Judicial rulings in vaccine-injury cases found manufacturers liable, not for the sale of products carrying a risk of inflicting harm, but rather for failing to inform vaccine recipients of the dangers. These developments have been consistent with the renewed emphasis in American culture since the 1960s and 1970s on the rights of the individual and his or her prerogative to choose.[23]

Tension between informed consent and lesser harms can be understood in terms of conflicting principles—autonomy, on the one hand, and nonmaleficence and beneficence, on the other—that have been central to the thinking of American bioethicists. In the late 1970s, Tom Beauchamp and James Childress, philosophers at Georgetown University's Kennedy Institute, sought to systematize bioethics by formulating principles that could be applied to cases. In *Principles of Biomedical Ethics,* they articulated four such notions: autonomy, nonmaleficence, beneficence, and justice. While "principlism" has had its critics, many within the field of bioethics quickly adopted it as the standard approach to decision making. And while Beauchamp and Childress intended the four tenets to have equal weight in the consideration of bioethical dilemmas, autonomy quickly emerged as dominant. It became the default invoked when principles conflicted. I have already noted that trends in American culture and jurisprudence have supported the preeminent position of autonomy in the ethos of American bioethics. Paul Wolpe, commenting on the "triumph of autonomy," suggests there are other reasons for this dominance as well. The individual's right to decide is a relatively straightforward concept. But the meanings of nonmaleficence, beneficence, and justice are slippery and open to multiple constructions in particular cases. "Of the four principles," Wolpe writes, "only autonomy is easily codified into a set of rules and regulations."[24] And codified it is. The result is a highly elaborated set of guidelines for securing the informed consent of patients and research subjects.

Arguably, our present regulatory environment has moved too far in embracing individual autonomy—and its implementation through consent procedures—and too far away from holding researchers accountable for protecting subjects from harm greater than that posed by their underlying disease. The author of a recent editorial on the Penn OTC trials comments that "one of the most important lessons" from the experiment "is that ethics committees can give too much weight to ensuring informed consent and not enough attention to minimizing the harm associated with participation in research."[25] The preeminence of autonomy has ironic consequences that have received insufficient attention in the literature on bioethics and human-subjects regulation. Subjects' consent serves to legitimize the conduct of hazardous experiments and to relieve investigators of legal, if not moral, responsibility for subsequent human injury. After all, should researchers be held culpable if subjects were fully informed and freely chose to assume the hazards? In short, informed consent has served to shift the burden of risk assumption from the researchers initiating an experiment and the broader research community to the subjects of biomedical research.

Expecting Miracles

A final set of issues relate to features of the cultural environment of research oversight that regulatory bodies have been poorly equipped to address. Quite frequently, some researchers promote, and lay constituencies hold, unrealistic notions about the speed with which innovations can be developed and safely introduced into clinical practice. Such expectations influence risk-benefit calculations and help fuel a rush into human trials.

Gene therapy is a field in which unrealistic hopes about the pace of clinical progress has been widespread. After Gelsinger's death, LeRoy Walters, the Kennedy Institute bioethicist who headed the RAC for many years, expressed disappointment that gene-transfer trials had not yielded better outcomes for patients. "If someone had told us in 1990 that after 300 studies in the United States alone, there will be only five or ten patients that you can point to who've benefited from gene transfer techniques, we would have thought that that's much too pessimistic a projection. But that's what, in fact, has happened."[26] At least some scientists have been less surprised by this course of events. Richard Mulligan observes that, "from the beginning," gene therapy "was overhyped, overpromised, oversold—expected to provide miracles on demand."[27] In the mid-1990s, Harold Varmus convened a panel to evaluate the NIH's investment in gene-transfer research. The panel's report appeared within days of the RAC's approval of Wilson's OTC protocol. Its authors, Stuart Orkin and Arno Motulsky, wrote that "overselling of the results of laboratory and clinical studies by investigators and their sponsors . . . has lead to the mistaken and widespread perception that gene therapy is further developed and more successful than it actually is." Orkin and Motulsky pointed to unsolved problems in all aspects of the field, including "shortcomings in all gene transfer vectors and an inadequate understanding of the biological interaction of these vectors with the host."[28]

Excessive optimism about the pace at which laboratory medicine will yield clinical advances is by no means unusual. Initial stages in the development of numerous medical interventions have been marked by disheartening human applications. Large numbers of deaths accompanied early vaccine testing. Observers critical of heroic clinical trials have described painful sequences of events surrounding experimentation with organ transplantation and with use of the Jarvis artificial heart.[29] The push to embark on hazardous—and often premature—human trials arises from multiple sources. Some critically ill patients are desperate for treatment and willing to find meaning in contributing to science. In recent years, patient groups have pressured federal agencies to make experimental therapies available as quickly as possible. Meanwhile, researchers and members of the broader public have been captivated by the power of scientific ideas. Deep-seated confidence in the therapeutic potential of medical science and associated technologies has a venerable history. The conviction that gene-transfer techniques would quickly yield safe and effective medical treatments is reminiscent of predictions, in the late nineteenth century, that vaccine breakthroughs were nearly in hand. Just after Robert Koch announced his discovery of the tuberculosis bacterium in 1882, newspapers in London and New York ran stories about the possibilities for a vaccine against tuberculosis. According to these accounts, it would be a matter of only a few years before a preventive intervention against tuberculosis would be available. In fact, four decades elapsed before researchers developed a tuberculosis vaccine appropriate for general use.[30]

What can be drawn from these observations about the design of research oversight? Are members of a research network likely to underestimate the risks of human experiments undertaken in their area of study? Is placing the assessment of research hazards in the hands of such specialists the equivalent of assigning to foxes the job of guarding the henhouse? I think the analogy is inapt. Optimism about the pace of medical advance goes well beyond members of the scientific community; it is a feature of the cultural context of clinical research. Furthermore, scientific experts differ substantially in their estimates of research hazards and in their degree of risk tolerance. When compared to clinical investigators, laboratory researchers are often more skeptical of claims about likely therapeutic benefits, as well as more averse to proceeding with clinical trials before scientific problems are adequately solved at the bench. The implication of the preceding discussion for regulatory policy is this: effective management of expert oversight of investigatory hazards requires care in the selection of scientific reviewers. Which investigators are chosen to serve on scientific oversight panels matters.

Lessons from the Past

I have argued that an optimally designed system for regulating human-subjects research would make judicious use of the scientific community's expertise and indigenous morality. Researchers have longstanding traditions bearing on the conduct of human experiments, traditions that are an outgrowth, in large part, of the cognitive norms of science. Central among these is the logic of lesser harms. Networks of medical researchers have routinely examined evidence bearing on the safety and efficacy of experimental interventions, and have pressured members to stay within culturally prescribed bounds of risk. The constraints exercised by scientific problem groups are informal and highly imperfect. But it is possible to construct formal controls that marshal researchers' moral commitments and technical competencies. The scientific advisory panels used by some of the mid-twentieth-century organizations sponsoring medical research provide one example of how scientists' traditions have been effectively mobilized. These panels assigned judgments about risks to researchers with competencies in the relevant investigatory fields of inquiry. Designed in this manner, research oversight fostered the flow of information bearing on experimental hazards among members of scientific problem groups.

It is the expert in a specialized investigatory field, drawing upon findings from that arena of study, who is best able to evaluate the hazards of human experiments. Such scientists are cognizant of professional practices specific to investigatory fields that bear on the management of investigatory hazards. Researchers' competencies and familiarity with indigenous morality remain crucial resources in the design of formal research oversight. Centralized panels of scientific specialists remain a viable model for how the use of expert knowledge might be organized.

The dangers of human experiments cannot always be anticipated, nor can research accidents always be prevented. But today's regulatory arrangements leave considerable room for improvement. Our current system of IRBs fails to utilize effectively either the research community's expertise or its traditions for containing investigatory hazards. Committees drawn from one institution and a broad range of research fields lack the knowledge to make informed judgments about the hazards of many of the protocols under their review. Local review boards have been more effective in implementing procedures for securing the consent of human subjects. But consent in the absence of adequate controls over risks has poorly understood consequences. It serves to shift the burden of risk assumption from researchers and the scientific community to the subjects of human experiments.

Prospects for the Future

Researchers' ability to evaluate the risks and benefits of human experiments rests in part on their expertise and skills. It relies also on the free flow of information among members of scientific problem groups. Academically based medical investigators have routinely shared research materials, laboratory techniques, and reports on the outcome of empirical studies. Sociologists consider such patterns to be a feature of the gift culture of science—a culture in which researchers contribute their discoveries to the scientific community, in return for the recognition of peers.[31] But the appearance of new types of corporate sponsorship of university-based clinical research is now threatening to undermine both cooperative exchanges among medical researchers and the unimpeded flow of information bearing on investigatory hazards.

Until recently, the distinction between industry and academic research was fairly clear-cut. Some university-based investigators conducted research under contract with pharmaceutical or equipment companies, but few had a direct financial interest in the products being developed or tested. If an occasional investigator withheld information about the outcome of research at the behest of a corporate sponsor, this was not a common practice among academic scientists. However, since the 1980s, new forms of entrepreneurialism have emerged in the biotechnology sector. Two developments have helped spur their appearance: court rulings allowing gene sequences, proteins, cells, and other biological materials to be patented and federal legislation encouraging private development of products resulting from publicly funded research.[32] Aided by these trends in public policy, academic medical investigators have been establishing their own firms to capitalize on the commercial potential of their research findings. Many of the universities employing these scientists have become equity partners in the firms, giving the academic institutions a financial interest in the companies.[33] Meanwhile, the investigators and universities are eligible for federal research support for experiments aimed at developing and testing commercially viable biological techniques and products.

Such corporate arrangements have been widespread among gene-therapy researchers. W. French Anderson, who in 1990 spearheaded the first RAC-approved gene-transfer trial, created the venture capital–funded firm Genetic Therapy, Inc., in 1986. Other scientists initiating early gene-therapy trials also sought corporate backing. In 1992, three groups won RAC approval to proceed with human experiments. The leader of each either founded a new biotechnology company or forged a partnership with an existing firm. Ronald Crystal established Gen Vec. Michael Welsh collaborated with Genzyme. James Wilson created Genova.[34] These companies have provided scientists with funding, managed patents, and planned for the manufacture and sale of genetically engineered products. Genova provided about a quarter of the budget for Wilson's Institute for Human Gene Therapy. The profits accruing from even undeveloped biotechnology patents have been considerable. In the aftermath of the Penn OTC experiment, managers of Genova sold the company in a deal worth $90 million. Wilson's share of the sale was valued at $13.5 million.[35]

Critics of the new corporate arrangements point out that conflicts of interest arise in handling research subjects when investigators have a financial stake in the results of their research. Some argue that scientists with equity holdings in research products may be willing to expose human subjects to high levels of risk in pursuit of monetary gain. Discussion at the February 2000 congressional hearings that examined Jesse Gelsinger's death underscored this possibility. "At the Hearings," one observer reports, "the doctors at the University of Pennsylvania . . . were depicted, in effect, as rogues willing to cut corners and sacrifice trusting patients in the race for fame, glory and biomedical riches."[36] Commentators who discuss entrepreneurialism in medical science emphasize conflicts of interest and typically recommend that researchers be required to disclose their financial holdings in consent documents read and signed by subjects.[37] A growing literature on conflicts of interest in clinical research has emerged since the mid-1990s. Recent reports from the Association of American Medical Colleges acknowledge dilemmas created by entrepreneurial arrangements for both individual researchers and academic institutions. The association recommends procedures for both disclosure and conflict-of-interest review.[38] But such procedural responses are unlikely to fully protect subjects from corporate incursions in science or to address the full range of problems that these incursions create.

The perspective of this book suggests that one of the most corrosive effects of entrepreneurialism in medical research may be its impact on the gift culture of science. The outcome may be that researchers come to behave more like isolated entrepreneurs than members of a scientific community. The norm of contributing discoveries in exchange for the recognition of peers is not one that prevails among industry competitors. Academic researchers with financial ties to biotech firms may decline to engage in some cooperative exchanges lest a competitor gain advantage. They may be reluctant to report negative outcomes or adverse events, least their stock values fall. If the competitive nature of scientific entrepreneurialism significantly undermines the flow of information within colleague networks, researchers' ability to assess the risks entailed in human experiments will be seriously compromised. With the advent of this new corporate environment in medical science, it is more important than ever that federal oversight agencies actively promote the open dissemination of findings bearing on the risks of human experiments.

Notes

Record Groups and Repositories

AFEB Records

Office of the Executive Secretary, Armed Forces Epidemiology Board, Interservice Agencies, Record Group 334, National Archives and Records Administration, College Park, Md.

AV Papers

Antivivisection Papers, Record Group 600–1, Rockefeller University Archives, Rockefeller Archive Center, Sleepy Hollow, N.Y.

Business Manager's Files

Business Manager's Subject Files, Rockefeller Institute, Record Group 210.3, Rockefeller University Archives, Rockefeller Archive Center, Sleepy Hollow, N.Y.

Commissioner's Files

Health Commissioner's Files, New York City Municipal Archives

DRL Records

Dermatological Research Laboratory, College of Physicians of Philadelphia

Flexner Papers

Simon Flexner Papers, American Philosophical Society, Philadelphia

Francis Papers

Thomas Francis Jr. Papers, Michigan Historical Collection, Bentley Historical Library, University of Michigan, Ann Arbor

Meyer Papers

Karl F. Meyer Papers, Bancroft Library, University of California, Berkeley

NFIP Materials

National Foundation for Infantile Paralysis, Cincinnati Medical Heritage Center, University of Cincinnati

NFIP Records

National Foundation for Infantile Paralysis, March of Dimes, White Plains, N.Y.

NIH Records

National Institutes of Health, Record Group 443, National Archives and Records Administration, College Park, Md.

NIH-OD Files

National Institutes of Health, Office of the Director, Subject Files, 1950–82, National Institutes of Health, Bethesda, Md.

NYF Records

New York Foundation Records, New York Foundation, New York City

OSG Records

Office of the Surgeon General, U.S. Army, Record Group 112, National Archives and Records Administration College Park, Md.

OSRD Records

Office of Scientific Research and Development, Record Group 227, National Archives and Records Administration, College Park, Md.

PBBC Records

President's Birthday Ball Commission, Franklin D. Roosevelt Library, Hyde Park, N.Y.

PEB Clipping Collection

Philadelphia Evening Bulletin Newsclipping Collection, Temple University Urban Archives, Philadelphia

PHS Records

U.S. Public Health Service, Record Group 90, National Archives and Records Administration, College Park, Md.

RAC Records

Recombinant DNA Advisory Committee, Office of Recombinant DNA Activities, now the Office of Biotechnology Activities, National Institutes of Health, Bethesda, Md.

Reports to RIMR Scientific Directors

Reports to the Board of Scientific Directors of the Rockefeller Institute for Medical Research, Record Group 439, Rockefeller University Archives, Rockefeller Archive Center, Sleepy Hollow, N.Y.

RF Project Files

Grants Administration Files, Rockefeller Foundation, Record Group 1.1, Projects, Rockefeller Foundation Archives, Rockefeller Archive Center, Sleepy Hollow, N.Y.

Rivers Papers

Thomas Rivers Papers, American Philosophical Society, Philadelphia

Rous Papers

Peyton Rous Papers, American Philosophical Society, Philadelphia

Sabin Papers

Albert Sabin Papers, Cincinnati Medical Heritage Center, University of Cincinnati

Salk Papers

Jonas Salk Papers, Mandeville Special Collections Library, University of California, San Diego

Stokes Papers

Joseph Stokes Jr. Papers, American Philosophical Society, Philadelphia

Introduction

1. Accounts of the creation of federal human-subjects regulations in the United States include William C. Curran, "Government Regulation of the Use of Human Subjects in Medical Research: The Approach of Two Federal Agencies," in *Experimentation with Human Subjects*, ed. Paul A. Freund (New York: George Braziller, 1970), pp. 402–53; Ruth R. Faden and Tom L. Beauchamp, *A History and Theory of Informed Consent* (New York: Oxford University Press, 1986); Mark S. Frankel, "The Development of Policy Guidelines Governing Human Experimentation in the United States: A Case Study of Public Policy-Making for Science and Technology," *Ethics in Science and Medicine* 2 (1975): 43–59; Mark. S. Frankel, "Public Policy Making for Biomedical Research: The Case of Human Experimentation" (Ph.D. diss., George Washington University, 1976). Robert J. Levine notes that the term "institutional review board" came into use in 1974 with passage of the National Research Act. See "Ethical Practices, Institutional Oversight, and Enforcement," in *International Encyclopedia of the Social and Behavioral Sciences*, ed. Neil J. Smelser and P. B. Baltes (New York: Elsevier, 2001), pp. 4770–74. For discussion of bioethics commissions convened in the 1970s and 1980s, see Dan W. Brock, "Public Policy and Bioethics," in *Encyclopedia of Bioethics*, ed. Warren T. Reich (New York: Free Press, 1995), 4:2181–87; Bradford H. Gray, "Bioethics Commissions: What Can We Learn from Past Successes and Failures?" in *Society's Choices: Social and Ethical Decision Making in Biomedicine*, ed. Ruth E. Bulger, Elizabeth M. Bobby, and Harvey V. Fineberg (Washington D.C.: National Academy Press, 1995), pp. 261–306; and Albert R. Jonsen, *The Birth of Bioethics* (New York: Oxford University Press, 1998). Robert J. Levine elaborates the standards embedded in federal regulatory codes in *Ethics and Regulation of Clinical Research* (Baltimore: Urban & Schwarzenberg, 1986).

2. On the consolidation of bioethics as a scholarly field and policy arena in the 1970s, consult Renée C. Fox, "The Evolution of American Bioethics: A Sociological Perspective," in *Social Science Perspectives on Medical Ethics*, ed. George Weisz (Dordrecht: Kluwer, 1990), pp. 201–17; Jonsen, *Birth of Bioethics;* Albert R. Jonsen and Andrew Jameton, "History of Medical Ethics: The United States in the Twentieth Century," in Reich, *Encyclopedia of Bioethics*, 3:1616–32; David J. Rothman, "Human Experimentation and the Origins of Bioethics in the United States," in Weisz, *Social Science Perspectives on Medical Ethics*, pp. 185–200; David J. Rothman, *Strangers at the Bedside: A History of How Law and Bioethics Transformed Medical Decision Making* (New York: Basic Books, 1991); M. L. Tina Stevens, *Bioethics in America: Origins and Cultural Politics* (Baltimore: Johns Hopkins University Press, 2000). Paul Starr develops the notion of the generalization of rights in *The Social Transformation of American Medicine* (New York: Basic Books, 1982). Faden and Beauchamp discuss court rulings that defined the meaning of informed consent in *History and Theory of Informed Consent*. On the Nuremberg codes of the late 1940s, see George J. Annas and Michael A. Grodin, eds., *Nazi Doctors and the Nuremberg Code* (New York: Oxford University Press, 1992); Jon H. Harkness, "Research behind Bars: A History of Nontherapeutic Re-

search on American Prisoners" (Ph.D. diss., University of Wisconsin, Madison, 1996); Paul M. McNeill, *The Ethics and Politics of Human Experimentation* (Cambridge: Cambridge University Press, 1993). While policy advocates drew on the Nuremberg codes in the 1960s, several authors comment that, in the postwar era, American investigators viewed the codes as having little relevance to their own research activities. See Advisory Committee on Human Radiation Experiments, *Final Report* (Washington, D.C.: U.S. Government Printing Office, 1995), p. 151; Rothman, *Strangers at the Bedside*, pp. 62–63.

3. Henry K. Beecher, "Ethics and Clinical Research," *New England Journal of Medicine* 74 (1966): 1354–60.

4. Renée C. Fox and Judith P. Swazey also distinguish medical morality and medical ethics in "Medical Morality Is Not Bioethics: Medical Ethics in China and the United States," *Perspectives in Biology and Medicine* 27, no. 3 (spring 1984): 336–360. Other work elaborating medical morality includes Robert Baker, ed., *The Codification of Medical Morality*, vol. 2, *Anglo-American Medical Ethics and Medicine Jurisprudence in the Nineteenth Century* (Dordrecht: Kluwer, 1995); Robert Baker, Dorothy Porter, and Roy Porter, eds., *The Codification of Medical Morality*, vol. 1, *Medical Ethics and Etiquette in the Eighteenth Century* (Dordrecht: Kluwer, 1993); Stanley Joel Reiser, Arthur J. Dyck, and William J. Curran, eds., *Ethics in Medicine: Historical Perspectives and Contemporary Concerns* (Cambridge: MIT Press, 1977). On the moral oversight of clinical research in Europe before and after formal regulation, see Ulrich Tröhler and Stella Reiter-Theil, eds., *Ethical Codes in Medicine: Foundations and Achievements of Codification since 1947* (Aldershot, England: Ashgate, 1998), and Ulrich Tröhler, "Human Research: From Ethos to Law, from National to International Regulation," in *Historical and Philosophical Perspectives on Biomedical Ethics: From Paternalism to Autonomy?* ed. Andreas-Holger Maehle and Johanna Geyer-Kordesch, pp. 95–118 (Aldershot, England: Ashgate, 2002).

5. Susan E. Lederer, *Subjected to Science: Human Experimentation in America before the Second World War* (Baltimore: Johns Hopkins University Press, 1995), pp. xv–xvi.

6. William Osler, "The Evolution of the Idea of Experiment in Medicine," *Transactions of the Congress of American Physicians and Surgeons* 7 (1907): 7–8.

7. Martin S. Pernick, "The Patient's Role in Medical Decisionmaking: A Social History of Informed Consent in Medical Therapy," in *Making Health Care Decisions*, vol. 3, ed. President's Commission for the Study of Ethical Problems in Medicine and Biomedical and Behavioral Research (Washington, D.C.: U.S. Government Printing Office, 1982), p. 3.

8. On debate over Pernick's claims regarding consent, see Faden and Beauchamp, *History and Theory of Informed Consent;* Jay Katz, *The Silent World of Doctor and Patient* (New York: Free Press, 1984); Wendy Mariner, "Informed Consent in the Post-Modern Era," *Law and Social Inquiry* 13, no. 2 (1988): 385–406.

9. Lederer, *Subjected to Science*, p. 9. Early rules for securing consent are discussed also in the Advisory Committee on Human Radiation Experiments, *Final Report*, chaps. 1 and 2.

10. Martin S. Pernick, *A Calculus of Suffering: Pain, Professionalism, and Anesthesia in Nineteenth Century America* (New York: Columbia University Press, 1985), p. 99–101. Other accounts attributing probabilistic reasoning among American physicians to the influence of Louis and the Paris school include Erwin H. Ackerknecht, *Medicine at the Paris Hospital, 1794–1848* (Baltimore: Johns Hopkins University Press, 1967); William Osler, "The Influence of Louis on American Medicine," in *An Alabama Student, and Other Biographical*

Essays (New York: Oxford University Press, 1908), pp. 189–210; Richard H. Shryock, "The History of Quantification in Medical Science," *Isis* 52, part 2 (June 1961): 215–37. Recent scholarship points to the application of quantitative reasoning in eighteenth-century Britain not only in matters related to smallpox inoculation—as discussed in chapter 1— but also to medical therapeutics more broadly. See Ulrich Tröhler, "*To Improve the Evidence of Medicine": The Eighteenth Century British Origins of a Critical Approach* (Edinburgh: College of Physicians of Edinburgh, 2000).

11. Pernick, *Calculus of Suffering*, pp. 93–124. Quotation from American Medical Association, "Report of the Committee on Surgery," *Transactions of the American Medical Association*, April 1852, p. 450.

12. Renée C. Fox, and Judith P. Swazey, *Courage to Fail: A Social View of Organ Transplants and Dialysis* (1974; Chicago: University of Chicago Press, 1978), p. 66.

13. Joseph Fletcher, "Our Shameful Waste of Human Tissue: An Ethical Problem for the Living and the Dead," in *The Religious Situation, 1969*, ed. Donald R. Cutler (Boston: Beacon Press, 1969), pp. 236.

14. Harry M. Marks, "Where Do Ethics Come From? The Case of Human Experimentation" (paper delivered at the Center for Biomedical Ethics, Case Western Reserve University, Cleveland, March 1988). One implication of the link between the character of science and research morality is that methodological innovations can create new moral dilemmas. On moral issues accompanying the advent of randomized clinical trials, see, for example, Austin Bradford Hill, "Medical Ethics and Controlled Clinical Trials," in *Clinical Investigation in Medicine: Legal, Ethical, and Moral Aspects*, ed. Irving Ladimer and Roger Newman (Boston: Boston University Law-Medicine Research Institute, 1963), pp. 370–83; Kenneth F. Schaffner, "Ethical Problems in Clinical Trials," *Journal of Medicine and Philosophy* 11 (1986): 297–315; and Harry M. Marks, *The Progress of Experiment: Science and Therapeutic Reform in the United States, 1900–1990* (Cambridge: Cambridge University Press, 1997).

15. David D. Rutstein, "The Ethical Design of Human Experiments," in Freund, *Experimentation with Human Subjects*, p. 384. Conversely, that properly executed science contributes to the solution of social problems was a longstanding and widely held notion. See David A. Hollinger, "Inquiry and Uplift: Late Nineteenth Century American Academics and the Moral Efficiency of Scientific Practice," in *The Authority of Experts: Studies in History and Theory*, ed. Thomas L. Haskell (Bloomington: Indiana University Press, 1984), pp. 142–56.

16. Osler, "Evolution of the Idea of Experiment in Medicine," p. 7.

17. Francis D. Moore, "Therapeutic Innovation: Ethical Boundaries in the Initial Clinical Trials of New Drugs and Surgical Procedures," in Freund, *Experimentation with Human Subjects*, p. 367. Fox and Swazey address the moral status of animal experimentation in *Courage to Fail*, pp. 69–70.

18. On moratoria in the performance of mitral-valve surgery, artificial heart implants, and a variety of transplant procedures, see, respectively, Judith Swazey and Renée C. Fox, "The Clinical Moratorium: A Case Study of Mitral Valve Surgery," in Freund, *Experimentation with Human Subjects*, pp. 315–57; Fox and Swazey, *Courage to Fail*; and Renée C. Fox and Judith P. Swazey, *Spare Parts: Organ Replacement in American Society* (New York: Oxford University Press, 1992). Diana B. Dutton discusses a moratorium in recombinant DNA trials in *Worse than the Disease: Pitfalls of Medical Progress* (New York: Cambridge University Press, 1988).

19. Lawrence K. Altman, *Who Goes First? The Story of Self-Experimentation in Medicine* (New York: Random House, 1986).

20. Osler, "Evolution of the Idea of Experiment in Medicine," p. 8. Lederer's observations on the public relations value of self-experimentation are found in *Subjected to Science*, p. 137.

21. Advisory Committee on Human Radiation Experiments, *Final Report*, pp. 137–38. Rothman notes that World War II researchers "who understood the need to make subjects' participation informed and voluntary" in some experiments also found it "easy to disregard the requirements" in other clinical studies (*Strangers at the Bedside*, p. 48).

22. Discussing other arenas of social life, Aaron V. Cicourel notes that how a norm fits particular situations is a matter of judgment. See "Basic and Normative Rules in the Negotiation of Status and Role," in *Studies in Social Interaction*, ed. David Sudnow (New York: Free Press, 1972), pp. 229–58.

23. Fox and Swazey, *Courage to Fail*, pp. 60–83. Medical researchers have offered another reason why experiments and therapy are difficult to distinguish. When defending human experimentation, they have routinely argued that clinical practice is itself an experiment. Thus, William Osler remarks, "Each dose of medicine given is an experiment, as it is impossible to predict in every instance what the result will be" ("Evolution of the Idea of Experiment in Medicine," p. 7). This echoes earlier statements made by American clinician Oliver Wendell Holmes in 1884 and by the French experimental physiologist Claude Bernard in 1865: "Every administration of a remedy is an experiment" (Oliver Wendell Holmes, "Experiments in Medicine," *Boston Medical and Surgical Journal* 30 [April 10, 1884]: 202). "Physicians make therapeutic experiments daily on their patients" (Claude Bernard, *An Introduction to the Study of Experimental Medicine* [1865; New York: Dover, 1957], p. 101).

24. Pernick notes the persistence of debate over the priority of common versus individual good (*Calculus of Suffering*, p. 124).

25. On uncertainties in medical practice, see Renée C. Fox, "Training for Uncertainty," in *The Student Physician*, ed. Robert K. Merton, George G. Reader, and Patricia L. Kendall (Cambridge: Harvard University Press, 1957), pp. 207–41; Renée C. Fox, "The Evolution of Medical Uncertainty," *Milbank Memorial Fund Quarterly* 58, no. 1 (1980): 1–49; Donald Light, "Uncertainty and Control in Professional Training," *Journal of Health and Social Behavior* 6 (1979): 141–51. Susan Leigh Star addresses varieties of uncertainty in biomedical research in "Scientific Work and Uncertainty," *Social Studies of Science* 15 (1985): 391–427.

26. On negotiations over the meaning of empirical findings, see, for example, Nigel G. Gilbert, "The Transformation of Research Findings into Scientific Knowledge," *Social Studies of Science* 6 (1976): 281–306; and Star, "Scientific Work and Uncertainty."

27. Bernard Barber et al., *Research on Human Subjects: Problems of Social Control in Medical Experimentation* (New Brunswick: Transaction Books, 1979). These authors also discuss professional and organizational stances toward research ethics but their reliance on survey data limits the scope of their institutional analysis.

28. The literature on problem groups includes Belver C. Griffith and Nicholas C. Mullins, "Coherent Social Groups in Scientific Change," *Science* 117 (1972): 959–64; Michael J. Mulkay, G. Nigel Gilbert, and Steve Woolgar, "Problem Areas and Research Networks in Science," *Sociology* 9 (1975): 187–203. On gift culture among and exchanges

within research communities, see Warren O. Hagstrom, *The Scientific Community* (New York: Basic Books, 1965); Adele E. Clarke, "Research Materials and Reproductive Science in the United States, 1910–1940," in *Physiology in the American Context, 1985–1940*, ed. Gerald Geison. (Bethesda: American Philosophical Society, 1987), pp. 323–50; Harry M. Marks, "Local Knowledge: Experimental Communities and Experimental Practices, 1918–1950" (paper delivered at the Conference on Twentieth-Century Health Science, University of California, San Francisco, May 1988).

29. Graham S. Wilson, *The Hazards of Immunization* (London: Athlone Press, 1967).

30. Rabies and some AIDS vaccines are exceptions to this statement. These immunizing agents are administered after exposure to disease but before the appearance of clinical symptoms.

31. Overviews of the history of vaccination include Susan L. Plotkin and Stanley A. Plotkin, "A Short History of Vaccination," in *Vaccines*, ed. Stanley A. Plotkin and Walter A. Orenstein (Philadelphia: Saunders, 1999), pp. 1–12; Stanley A. Plotkin and Susan L. Plotkin, "Vaccination: One Hundred Years Later," in *World's Debt to Pasteur*, ed. Hilary Koprowsky and Stanley A. Plotkin (New York: Liss, 1985), pp. 83–106; H. J. Parish, *History of Immunization* (London: Livingstone, 1965).

32. Studies pointing to the importance of organizational processes to moral decision making in clinical settings include Renée R. Anspach, *Deciding Who Lives: Fateful Choices in the Intensive-Care Nursery* (Berkeley and Los Angeles: University of California Press, 1993); Charles L. Bosk, *All God's Mistakes: Genetic Counseling in a Pediatric Hospital* (Chicago: University of Chicago Press, 1992); Daniel F. Chambliss, *Beyond Caring: Hospitals, Nurses, and the Social Organization of Ethics* (Chicago: University of Chicago Press, 1996); Carol A. Heimer and Lisa R. Staffen, *For the Sake of the Children: The Social Organization of Responsibility in the Hospital and the Home* (Chicago: University of Chicago Press, 1998); Robert Zussman, *Intensive Care: Medical Ethics and the Medical Profession* (Chicago: University of Chicago Press, 1992). Early sociological studies of medical decision making include Renée C. Fox, *Experiment Perilous* (Glencoe, Ill.: Free Press, 1959); and Diana Crane, *The Sanctity of Life* (New York: Russell Sage, 1975). For commentaries on sociological perspectives on bioethics, see Renée C. Fox, "The Sociology of Bioethics," in *The Sociology of Medicine: A Participant Observer's View* (Englewood Cliffs, N.J.: Prentice-Hall, 1989), pp. 224–76; Daniel F. Chambliss, "Is Bioethics Irrelevant?" *Contemporary Sociology* 22: 5 (1993): 649–52; Raymond DeVries and Janardan Subedi, eds., *Bioethics and Society: Constructing the Ethical Enterprise* (Upper Saddle River, N.J.: Prentice-Hall, 1998); Barry C. Hoffmaster, ed., *Bioethics in Social Context* (Philadelphia: Temple University Press, 2001); Robert Zussman, "Sociological Perspectives on Medical Ethics and Decision-Making," *Annual Review of Sociology* 23 (1997): 171–89.

33. Historians of medical science have commented on the research community's concern with social legitimacy in general and public reactions to investigatory hazards in particular. Lederer remarks that, in the years between the two world wars, it was concern with the community's social standing that motivated research leaders to insist "that consent (or parental permission) and avoidance of risk were essential conditions of ethical human experimentation." They did so "to minimize the potential loss of public support" in the face of antivivisection protests (*Subjected to Science*, p. 125). Both Marks and Rothman note that World War II researchers were alert to public responses to hazardous experiments. In "Where Do Ethics Come From?" Marks recounts explicit discussion of the potential for "ad-

verse public reaction" in 1942–43 debates among scientific leaders over the conduct of an experiment to test the effectiveness of chemical treatment of gonorrhea that involved infecting subjects with the disease. Rothman suggests that wartime researchers were careful about securing consent when they thought public scrutiny of their work was likely (*Strangers at the Bedside*, p. 48).

Chapter One

1. For one account of tensions between medical researchers and clinicians, see Gerald L. Geison, "Divided We Stand: Physiologists and Clinicians in the American Context," in *The Therapeutic Revolution: Essays in the Social History of American Medicine*, ed. Morris J. Vogel and Charles E. Rosenberg (Philadelphia: University of Pennsylvania, 1979), pp. 67–90.

2. I base my account of smallpox inoculation in early-eighteenth-century Europe largely on the work of Genevieve Miller and Andrea Rusnock, both of whom emphasize the role of scientific societies in the introduction of inoculation. Relevant publications by these authors include Genevieve Miller, *Adoption of Inoculation of Smallpox in England and France* (Philadelphia: University of Pennsylvania Press, 1957); Andrea A. Rusnock, "The Weight of Evidence and the Burden of Authority: Case Histories, Medical Statistics, and Smallpox Inoculation," in *Medicine in the Enlightenment*, ed. Roy Porter (Amsterdam: Rodopi Press, 1995), pp. 289–315; Andrea A. Rusnock, ed., *The Correspondence of James Jurin, 1684–1750: Physician and Secretary to the Royal Society* (Amsterdam: Rodopi Press, 1996); and Andrea A. Rusnock, *Vital Accounts: Quantifying Health and Population in Eighteenth-Century England and France* (Cambridge: Cambridge University Press, 2002). Other work on smallpox inoculation includes Peter Razell's *The Conquest of Smallpox: The Impact of Inoculation on Smallpox in Eighteenth Century Britain* (Sussex: Caliban Books, 1997) which points to widespread use of the procedure in late-eighteenth-century Britain.

3. Reports of smallpox deaths subsequent to inoculation further intensified public fears and inflamed the opposition. Not only were there occasional deaths among inoculated cases, but individuals with inoculated smallpox were contagious to those around them. Those contracting the disease after exposure to an inoculated individual were subject to the disease severity and mortality of natural smallpox. Opponents insisted that inoculation increased the severity of epidemics. Inoculators—largely surgeons—addressed the problem of contagion by recommending the isolation of patients in the weeks following the procedure.

4. The prisoners were released after the demonstration. None contracted smallpox subsequent to inoculation. The major primary source on the Newgate experiment is Charles Maitland, *Account of Inoculating the Smallpox* (London, 1722). Secondary accounts can be found in Miller, *Adoption of Inoculation of Smallpox in England and France*, and in C. W. Dixon, *Smallpox* (London: Churchill, 1962). Dixon describes the Newgate inoculations as the first planned experiment in immunology.

5. Jurin issued four editions of the pamphlet, *An Account of the Success of Inoculating the Smallpox in Great Britain*, one for each of the years 1724–27.

6. Rusnock elaborates Jurin's methods in "The Weight of Evidence and the Burden of Authority" and in *Vital Accounts*, pp. 49–66.

7. American physician Zabdiel Boylston provided reports to the Royal Society on the results of smallpox inoculation in Boston. Encouraged by the British inoculationists, Boyl-

ston published his *Historical Account of the Small-Pox Inoculated in New England* in 1726 and immediately presented a copy to the Royal Society. Miller discusses these events in *Adoption of Inoculation of Smallpox in England and France*. On the relation of inoculation use in America and Britain, see Genevieve Miller, "Smallpox Inoculation in England and America: A Reappraisal," *William and Mary Quarterly*, 3rd ser., 13, no. 4 (October 1956): 476–92.

8. J. G. Scheuchzer, *An Account of the Success of Inoculating the Smallpox in Great Britain for the Years 1727 and 1728* (London, 1929), p. 1729; Miller, *Adoption of Inoculation of Smallpox in England and France*, p. 121.

9. It was members of the upper strata who first adopted inoculation, and its early use occurred largely during epidemics. See Miller, *Adoption of Inoculation of Smallpox in England and France*, and Derrick Baxby, *Jenner's Smallpox Vaccine* (London: Heinemann, 1981).

10. Gerald L. Geison makes this point in "Pasteur's Work on Rabies: Reexamining the Ethical Issues," *Hastings Center Report* 8, no. 2 (1978): 26–33, and in *The Private Science of Louis Pasteur* (Princeton: Princeton University Press, 1995).

11. Discussion of early bills of mortality is found in Ian Hacking, *The Emergence of Probability* (London: Cambridge University Press, 1975), and in Rusnock, *Vital Accounts*, pp. 18–24. Hacking's book is a major source on the history of probability.

12. Steven Shapin, "Pump and Circumstance: Robert Boyle's Literary Technology," *Social Studies of Science* 14 (1984): 481–520; Steven Shapin and Simon Schaffer, *Leviathan and the Air-Pump: Hobbes, Boyle, and the Experimental Life* (Princeton: Princeton University Press, 1985).

13. Barbara J. Shapiro, *Probability and Certainty in Seventeenth Century Britain* (Princeton: Princeton University Press, 1983); Hacking, *Emergence of Probability*.

14. Miller, *Adoption of Inoculation of Smallpox in England and France*.

15. John Woodhouse to James Jurin, February 9, 1726, Royal Society, *Classified Papers* 23 (2), no. 90; cited in Rusnock, "The Weight of Evidence and the Burden of Authority," p. 303.

16. Commentaries on the public character of science in late-seventeenth- and early-eighteenth-century Britain include Jan Golinski, *Science as Public Culture: Chemistry and Enlightenment in Britain, 1760–1820* (New York: Cambridge University Press, 1992), and Larry R. Stewart, *The Rise of Public Science: Rhetoric, Technology, and Natural Philosophy in Newtonian Britain, 1660–1750* (Cambridge: Cambridge University Press, 1992).

17. Sources on the Bernoulli-D'Alembert controversy include Leslie Bradley, trans., *Smallpox Inoculation: An Eighteenth Century Mathematical Controversy* (Nottingham: University of Nottingham, 1971); Lorraine Daston, *Classical Probability in the Enlightenment* (Princeton: Princeton University Press, 1988); Thomas L. Haskins, *Jean d'Alembert: Science and the Enlightenment* (Oxford: Clarendon Press, 1970); Miller, *Adoption of Inoculation of Smallpox in England and France*; and Rusnock, *Vital Accounts*.

18. Miller, *Adoption of Inoculation of Smallpox in England and France*.

19. Many decades later, Simon Flexner made concessions to perceptions and preferences about risk when suggesting that an immune serum might be used during polio epidemics as an antidote to parental anxiety. In a paper published in 1928, Flexner describes results of laboratory experiments with monkeys suggesting that injections of convalescent serum might protect children against exposure to epidemic poliomyelitis. On the basis of

these tests, conducted on an unspecified number of animals, he and his collaborator "propose that convalescent human serum should be employed at times of stress and anxiety, when polio is epidemic, for producing passive immunization." They add: "We recognize that epidemic poliomyelitis is a disease of low incidence, and therefore the efficacy of the protective injections will not be easy to determine. We believe, however, that they may be used to diminish anxiety on the part of parents and others." See Simon Flexner and Fred W. Stewart, "Specific Prevention and Treatment of Epidemic Poliomyelitis," *New England Journal of Medicine* 199, no. 5 (August 2, 1928): 213–15.

20. Edward Jenner, *An Inquiry into the Causes and Effects of the Variolae Vaccinae* (1798; London: Dawsons, 1966).

21. Andrea Rusnock notes that William Woodville carried out vaccinations and inoculations on patients at the London Smallpox Hospital and, using the same method as Jurin, calculated ratios of deaths caused by each procedure. His initial conclusion, published in 1799, was that there was little to be gained from vaccination. Woodville would soon reverse his position on this matter (Andrea Rusnock, "Vaccination and the Evaluation of Risk" [paper delivered at the meetings of the American Association for the History of Medicine, Boston, May 2003]). T. H. Bradley reviewed contemporary experimental studies of inoculation and vaccination in "An Account of the Publications and Experiments on the Cow-Pox," *Medical and Physical Journal* 1, no. 1 (March 1799): 1–11. He compared the two procedures, arguing that inoculated smallpox carried a significant risk of mortality. In contrast, "the *natural* cow-pox has *never* proved fatal, and the vaccinated cow-pox was much milder than the natural" (emphasis in the original). It was reasonable to conclude, Bradley wrote, at this point quoting George Pearson, another early supporter of vaccination, that "there is great probability of the cow-pox [contracted through vaccination] either not proving fatal at all, or at most being much less frequently so, than the inoculated small-pox" (Pearson, *An Inquiry Concerning the History of the Cow Pox, Principally with a View to Supersede and Extinguish the Small Pox* [1798], p. 68). When endorsing vaccination, the Royal College of Physicians also compared the new procedure to inoculation: "Vaccination appears to be in general perfectly safe; instances to the contrary being extremely rare. The disease excited by it is slight, and seldom prevents those under its influence from following ordinary occupations. . . . It possesses material advantages over Inoculation for the Small Pox; which though productive of a disease generally mild, yet sometimes occasions alarming symptoms, and is in a few cases fatal" (Royal College of Physicians, *Report of the Royal College of Physicians of London on Vaccination* [London: Royal College of Physicians, 1807], pp. 3–4).

22. Cases of syphilis and erysipelas occasionally followed vaccination. Advocates for the procedure insisted that secondary infections resulted from passing lymph from patient to patient and could be prevented by using lymph from cows and by avoiding contaminated instruments.

23. The identity of the vaccinia virus was in contention for decades and is still undetermined. On this issue, see Baxby, *Jenner's Smallpox Vaccine*.

24. The secondary literature on debates over compulsory vaccination in Britain and on the political context in which they occurred includes Ann Beck, "Issues in the Anti-Vaccination Movement in England," *Medical History* 4, no. 4 (October 1960): 310–21; R. M. MacLeod, "Law, Medicine, and Public Opinion: The Resistance to Compulsory Health Legislation, 1870–1907," *Public Law*, summer 1967, pp. 107–28, and autumn 1967, pp. 189–210; Dorothy Porter and Roy Porter, "The Politics of Prevention: Anti-Vaccination and Pub-

lic Health in Nineteenth Century England, *Medical History* 32, no. 3 (July 1988): 231–52; Peter Baldwin, *Contagion and the State in Europe, 1830–1930* (Cambridge: Cambridge University Press, 1999).

25. Porter and Porter, "The Politics of Prevention," p. 243.

26. Anne Hardy, "Liberty, Equality, and Immunization: The English Experience since 1800" (paper delivered at the meetings of the American Association for the History of Medicine, Boston, May 2003).

27. Ibid., p. 4. On the declining incidence of smallpox in Britain, see Anne Hardy, *Epidemic Streets: Infectious Disease and the Rise of Preventive Medicine, 1856–1900* (Oxford: Clarendon Press, 1993).

28. Royal Commission on Vaccination, *A Report on Vaccination and its Results, Based on the Evidence Taken by the Royal Commission during the Years 1889–1897*, vol. 1, *Text of the Commission Report* (London: New Sydenham Society, 1898), p. 225.

29. Ibid., pp. 214–15.

30. Accompanying the *Times* editorial was a letter from British scientist John Tyndall, who used the occasion to reprehend the contemporary antivivisection movement. Tyndall extolled Koch's accomplishment and pointed out that it would not have been impossible without animal experimentation (*Times* [London], April 22, 1882, p. 11).

31. It was in the late 1920s that the Bacille Calmette-Guerin vaccine against tuberculosis was accepted for clinical use. See Kim Connelly Smith and Jeffrey R. Starke, "Bacille Calmette-Guerin Vaccine," in *Vaccines*, ed. Stanley A. Plotkin and Walter A. Orenstein (Philadelphia: Saunders, 1999), p. 119.

32. "Tubercular Disease," *Times* (London), April 22, 1882, p. 11; cited in Thomas D. Brock, *Robert Koch* (Madison: Science Tech, 1988), p. 131.

33. "The Tubercle Parasite," *New York Tribune*, May 3, 1882, p. 4. On the American press's intense interest in medical innovations beginning in the mid-1880s, see Bert Hansen, "America's First Medical Breakthrough: How Popular Excitement about French Rabies Cure in 1885 Raised New Expectations for Medical Progress," *American Historical Review* 103 (April 1998): 373–418; Bert Hansen, "New Images of a New Medicine: Visual Evidence for the Widespread Popularity of Therapeutic Discoveries in America after 1885," *Bulletin of the History of Medicine* 73, no. 4 (winter 1999): 629–78. On press coverage in France of Pasteur's anthrax experiments and the public framing there of debates over immunization, see Massimiano Bucchi, "The Public Science of Louis Pasteur: The Experiment on Anthrax Vaccine in the Popular Press of the Time," *History and Philosophy of the Life Sciences* 19 (1997): 181–209.

34. Geison reports that Pasteur actually treated two patients in May and June of 1885, before Meister and Jupille, but that he did not report these attempts to the scientific community. With the earlier patients—one of whom succumbed to rabies—Pasteur employed a different vaccine and immunization procedure than he used with Meister and Jupille. The earlier patients, Geison writes, "were treated by a method that had apparently never been successfully tested on animals with symptomatic rabies" (*Private Science of Louis Pasteur*, p. 204).

35. Rabies has a long incubation period. This makes it possible for individuals who have been exposed to the disease to acquire immunity from a vaccine if the immunizing agent is administered soon after exposure.

36. Geison describes the method Pasteur used with Meister. The immunizing agent
was composed of dried spinal marrow of rabbits that had succumbed to rabies. Meister received a series of thirteen injections over the course of ten days, each injection with a preparation that had been left to dry for a shorter time—and that was thus considered to be more
virulent the previous one. The final injection contained fresh spinal-cord tissue of a deceased rabies-infected rabbit—containing virus that had undergone serial passage through
rabbits (*Private Science of Louis Pasteur*, p. 215).

37. Ibid., p. 252.

38. Louis Pasteur, *Oeuvres de Pasteur*, ed. Pasteur Vallery-Radot, vol. 6 (Paris: Masson et
Cie, 1933), p. 591; cited in Geison, *Private Science of Louis Pasteur*, p. 232.

39. Geison, *Private Science of Louis Pasteur*, pp. 221–22.

40. Ibid., p. 240.

41. Ibid., pp. 221–22 and p. 337 n. 26.

42. René Dubos, *Louis Pasteur: Free Lance of Science* (New York: Charles Schribner,
1976), pp. 345–46.

43. Soon after Pasteur's rabies vaccine was introduced into general use, researchers became aware that, in a portion of recipients, the immunizing agent induced life-threatening
neuroparalysis—either during or just after the course of treatment. While rumors about
these incidents were widespread, there was, in Graham Wilson's words, "a conspiracy of si-
lence" at the Pasteur Institute about the preparation's side effects (*Hazards of Immunization* [London: Athlone Press, 1967], p. 180). In the 1920s, scientists began collecting and
publishing data on numbers of vaccine accidents per total vaccinations. Wilson writes that
one of the first compilations, published in 1927, estimated that there had been between 500
and 1,000 cases of vaccine induced neuropathology among 1,164,000 individuals treated
with Pasteur's vaccine (ibid., p. 181). Debate about Pasteur's vaccine was ongoing within
scientific circles during the late 1920s and early 1930s. Even today's rabies vaccines carry a
relatively high risk of serious neurological complications. For this reason, practitioners
avoid using them except in the event of known exposure.

44. Geison notes in *Private Science of Louis Pasteur* that the debates at the Académie de
Médecine did not attract attention from outside the professional community.

45. On the emergence of American laboratory medicine, see Joseph Ben-David, "Scientific Productivity and Academic Organization in Nineteenth Century Medicine," *American Sociological Review* 25, no. 6 (1960): 828–43.

46. Sources on the reform of medical education and creation of full-time faculty appointments include Sydney Halpern, "Professional Schools in the American University:
The Evolving Dilemma of Research and Practice," in *The Academic Profession: National, Disciplinary, and Institutional Settings*, ed. Burton R. Clark (Berkeley and Los Angeles: University of California Press, 1987), pp. 304–330.

47. My account of American antivivisectionism draws heavily on the work of Susan E.
Lederer, including *Subjected to Science: Human Experimentation in America before the Second
World War* (Baltimore: Johns Hopkins University Press, 1995); "The Controversy over Animal Experimentation in America, 1880–1914," in *Vivisection in Historical Perspective*, ed.
Nicolaas A. Rupke (London: Routledge, 1987), pp. 236–58; "Political Animals: The Shaping of Biomedical Research Literature in Twentieth-Century America," *Isis* 83, no. 1 (March
1992): 61–79. Also see Saul Benison, "In Defense of Medical Research," *Harvard Medical*

Alumni Bulletin 44 (1970): 16–23. Martin Kaufman notes that many antivivisectionists were also against compulsory vaccination ("The American Anti-Vaccinationists and Their Arguments," *Bulletin of the History of Medicine* 41 (1967): 463–79. For an international perspective on antivivisectionism, see Nicolaas A. Rupke, ed., *Vivisection in Historical Perspective* (London: Routledge, 1990).

48. Lederer, *Subjected to Science.*

49. Richard D. French, *Antivivisection and Medical Science in Victorian Society* (Princeton: Princeton University Press, 1975).

50. [Walter Cannon], "The Right and Wrong of Making Experiments on Human Beings," *JAMA* 67, no. 19 (November 4, 1916): 1372–73. On efforts by Cannon and others to counter antivivisectionist publicity and legislation, see Benison's "In Defense of Medical Research" and Lederer's "The Controversy over Animal Experimentation in America," "Political Animals," and *Subjected to Science.*

51. Richard M. Pearce, *The Charge of "Human Vivisection" as Presented in Antivivisection Literature*, Defense of Medical Research Pamphlet 26 (Chicago: Bureau on Protection of Medical Research, American Medical Association, 1914), p. 31.

52. Jay F. Schamberg, *Vaccination and Its Relation to Animal Experimentation*, Defense of Medical Research, Pamphlet 1 (Chicago: Bureau on Protection of Medical Research, American Medical Association, 1911), p. 43.

53. Ibid., p. 42.

54. On the transformation of the professions in the second half of the nineteenth and early decades of the twentieth century, see Samuel Haber, "The Professions and Higher Education in America: A Historical View," in *Higher Education and the Labor Market*, ed. Margaret S. Gordon (New York: Carnegie Foundation, 1974); Magali Sarfatti Larson, *The Rise of Professionalism: A Sociological Analysis* (Berkeley and Los Angeles: University of California Press, 1977). On the impact of scientific knowledge on medical practice in nineteenth-century America, see John Harley Warner, *The Therapeutic Perspective: Medical Practice, Knowledge, and Identity in America, 1820–1885* (Cambridge: Harvard University Press, 1986); Charles E. Rosenberg, "The Therapeutic Revolution: Medicine, Meaning, and Social Change in Nineteenth Century America," *Perspectives in Biology and Medicine* 20 (summer 1977): 485–506.

55. Lederer comments that self-experimentation "was an accepted feature of medical research in the mid-nineteenth century" (*Subjected to Science*, p. 18). Lawrence Altman points to several instances of self-experimentation during the seventeenth and eighteenth centuries. But most of his examples—there are dozens of them—occurred between the late nineteenth and mid-twentieth centuries (Lawrence K. Altman, *Who Goes First? The Story of Self-Experimentation in Medicine* [New York: Random House, 1987]). The great bulk of the vaccine trials that I discuss in chapters 2 and 3 of this volume began with self-experiments.

56. But researchers did include coded messages concerning the practice in their publications. Altman remarks that he culled much of his evidence for self-experimentation from "tables in the medical journal articles where the scientific data were listed case by case" (*Who Goes First?* p. 11). I found this type of evidence in a 1935 article by Thomas Francis Jr. describing an experiment in which human subjects received injections of live influenza virus. The paper included a table that listed each recipient, by initials, and the date of inocu-

lation. Francis's first human subject, inoculated three weeks before the others, bore the initials "T.F." (Thomas Francis Jr. and T. P. Magill, "Vaccination of Human Subjects with Virus of Human Influenza," *Proceedings of the Society for Experimental Biology and Medicine* 33, no. 4 [January 1936]: 606).

57. William Osler, "The Evolution of the Idea of Experiment in Medicine," *Transactions of the Congress of American Physicians and Surgeons* 7 (1907): 1–8.

58. Pearce, *The Charge of "Human Vivisection,"* pp. 29–30.

59. Altman, *Who Goes First?* p. 12.

60. Marie S. Winokur, superintendent of the Homewood School in the Germantown section of Philadelphia, wrote to Stokes about the status of his request to test a measles vaccine at the institution: "I have already spoken to the Chairman of my Health and Medical Committee and several Board Members about this, and the statement that you have inoculated your own child, has helped me convince them that this will not jeopardize our children's health." Winokur then addressed the problem of securing consent: "The fact that you have already inoculated your own child will aid me here too to get the consent of the children's parents, which I will have to procure before we can start this work." The Homewood School was a constituent of the Federation of Jewish Charities of Philadelphia. See Marie S. Winokur to Joseph Stokes Jr., November 7, 1940, Stokes Papers, box: Measles no. 5, folder: Squibb Institute no. 7.

61. In 1934, the Office of the U.S. Surgeon General asked two polio researchers— John Kolmer and William Park—to respond to complaints originating from antivivisectionists that one or both had tested experimental polio vaccines on orphans. In separate letters, the researchers acknowledged having used a new vaccine on children but portrayed the decision to do so as entirely appropriate. In justifying their actions, each pointed to the consent of the children's parents or guardians, prior animal testing, prior self-experimentation, and in the case of Kolmer, prior experiments with his own children. See John A. Kolmer to R. C. Williams, October 15, 1934, PHS Records, General Files, box 60, folder: Poliomyelitis. Park's letter is in the same folder.

62. Harry M. Marks, *The Progress of Experiment: Science and Therapeutic Reform in the United States, 1900–1990* (Cambridge: Cambridge University Press, 1997); Theodore M. Porter, *Trust in Numbers: The Pursuit of Objectivity in Science and Public Life* (Princeton: Princeton University Press, 1995); J. Rosser Matthews, *Quantification and the Quest for Medical Certainty* (Princeton: Princeton University Press, 1995).

63. David D. Rutstein, "The Ethical Design of Human Experiments," in *Experimentation with Human Subjects,* ed. Paul A. Freund (New York: George Braziller, 1970), p. 384.

64. In "Some Aspects of Cultural Growth in the Natural Sciences," *Social Research* 36 (1969): 22–52, Michael Mulkay argues that the core norms of the scientific community are technical in nature. Mulkay juxtaposes his position to that of Robert Merton, who, Mulkay argues, depicts the core norms of science as social in character. Merton's seminal statements on the cultural ethos of science include "Science and the Social Order" (1938) and "The Normative Structure of Science" (1942) in *The Sociology of Science,* ed. Normal W. Storer (Chicago: University of Chicago Press, 1973), pp. 254–66, 267–85. Other writers take issues with Mulkay's account of Merton's position. Harriet Zuckerman argues that Merton's work recognizes both cognitive and social norms in science. See Zuckerman's essay, "Deviant Behavior and Social Control in Science," in *Deviance and Social Change,* ed.

Edward Sagarin (Beverly Hills: Sage, 1977), pp. 87–138. And Nico Stehr notes that, in Merton's view, social norms of science are linked to its technical goals. Stehr's essay is "The Ethos of Science Revisited: Social and Cognitive Norms," *Sociological Inquiry* 48 (1978): 172–96.

65. Like other professional and institutional communities, scientific fields generate rich arrays of norms, ideologies, myths, symbols, and images. Scholars note that these ideational products have both internal and external functions. The culture of science promotes group cohesion by defining core tasks and purposes and by fostering agreements about the parameters of appropriate professional conduct. It also assists scientists in positioning themselves within the broader social order by justifying the group's claims to legitimacy, authority, and social resources. Warren O. Hagstrom discusses the varied purposes that disciplinary culture serves for emerging fields in *The Scientific Community* (New York: Basic Books, 1965).

66. Ann Swidler, "Culture in Action: Symbols and Strategies," *American Sociological Review* 51 (1986): 273–86.

Chapter Two

1. Literature on research networks includes Michael J. Mulkay, G. Nigel Gilbert, and Steve Woolgar, "Problem Areas and Research Networks in Science," *Sociology* 9 (1975): 187–203. On gift culture and exchanges within research communities, see Warren O. Hagstrom, *The Scientific Community* (New York: Basic Books, 1965); Adele E. Clarke, "Research Materials and Reproductive Science in the United States, 1910–1940," in *Physiology in the American Context, 1850–1940,* ed. Gerald Geison (Bethesda: American Philosophical Society, 1987), pp. 323–50.

2. Discussions of local knowledge among biological scientists include Susan Leigh Star, "Scientific Work and Uncertainty," *Social Studies of Science* 15 (1985): 391–427; and Harry M. Marks, "Local Knowledge: Experimental Communities and Experimental Practices, 1918–1950" (paper delivered at the Conference on Twentieth-Century Health Sciences, University of California, San Francisco, May 1988). Harry M. Collins examines the phenomenon among physical scientists in "The TEA Set: Tacit Knowledge and Scientific Networks," *Science Studies* 4 (1974): 165–86.

3. Clifford Geertz, *Local Knowledge* (New York: Basic Books, 1983), p. 4.

4. A number of scholars argue that the prestige system in professional and scientific communities provides a highly effective means for social control. On this viewpoint, see Hagstrom, *The Scientific Community,* and William Goode, "Community within a Community: The Professions," *American Sociological Review* 22 (1957): 194–200. In *Profession of Medicine* (New York: Harper and Row, 1970), Eliot Freidson identifies the colleague boycott as the principal means of social control within networks of physicians. He notes that ostracizing fails to protect the public because it does not remove poorly performing physicians from medical practice. Freidson also emphasizes that physicians are quite reluctant to impose even informal controls on colleagues. See, as well as *Profession of Medicine,* his *Doctoring Together* (New York: Elsevier, 1975). On the designation of outsiders as a means to enhance internal group cohesion, see Kai Erikson, *Wayward Puritans: A Study in the Sociology of Deviance* (New York: Wiley, 1966). For discussion of varieties of formal and informal control within medicine, see the introduction to Charles L. Bosk, *Forgive and Remember: Managing Medical Failure* (Chicago: University of Chicago Press, 1979).

5. I base my estimate of the number of polio researchers on International Committee for the Study of Infantile Paralysis, *Poliomyelitis* (Baltimore: Williams and Wilkins, 1932). This volume, prepared with funding from philanthropist Jeremiah Milbank, provides a comprehensive review of knowledge of infantile paralysis through the early 1930s. In its bibliography, approximately sixty American scientists appear as first authors of papers discussing laboratory studies of poliomyelitis. Another sixty or so American investigators— not in the previous group—appear as the second or third author on one or more papers describing laboratory research.

6. John R. Paul notes that, during the early decades of the twentieth century, the age distribution of polio cases shifted to include a higher portion of adults and older children. See *A History of Poliomyelitis* (New Haven: Yale University Press, 1971), pp. 346–47.

7. On public responses to epidemic poliomyelitis, see Naomi Rogers, *Dirt and Disease: Polio before FDR* (New Brunswick: Rutgers University Press, 1992), and Daniel J. Wilson, "A Crippling Fear: Experiencing Polio in the Era of FDR," *Bulletin of the History of Medicine* 72 (1998): 464–95. Statistics on polio cases in the 1916 epidemic are from Rogers, *Dirt and Disease*, p. 10.

8. Simon Flexner and Paul A. Lewis, "The Transmission of Acute Poliomyelitis to Monkeys," *JAMA* 53, no. 20 (November 13, 1909): 1639.

9. Discussion of expanding career tracks in medical research is found in Sydney A. Halpern, "Professional Schools in the American University: The Evolving Dilemma of Research and Practice," in *The Academic Profession: National, Disciplinary, and Institutional Settings*, ed. Burton R. Clark (Berkeley and Los Angeles: University of California Press, 1987), pp. 304–30; and Kenneth M. Ludmerer, *Learning to Heal: The Development of American Medical Education* (New York: Basic Books, 1985).

10. On early Rockefeller Foundation support for polio research, see "Infantile Paralysis: Summary," RF Project Files, series 200, box 25, folder 275: Infantile Paralysis, 1916–18. Milbank's support is described in International Committee for the Study of Infantile Paralysis, *Poliomyelitis*. On PBBC funding, see "The Medical Research Program of the National Foundation for Infantile Paralysis," a monograph prepared by the Historical Division, NFIP, August 1954, NFIP Materials, Cincinnati Medical Heritage Center. Also see "Special Report for the Information of Mr. Keith Morgan," PBBC Records, box 1: Correspondence and Reports of the Commission, section 16: Correspondence with Member of the Commission and the Medical Advisory Committee on the Report to Be Made to the President.

11. Sources on the early history of polio research include Saul Benison, "History of Polio Research in the United States: Appraisal and Lessons," in *The Twentieth-Century Sciences*, ed. Gerald Holton (New York: Norton, 1970), pp. 308–43; Saul Benison, "Poliomyelitis and the Rockefeller Institute: Social Effects and Institutional Response," *Journal of the History of Medicine* 29, no. 1 (January 1974): 74–92; Saul Benison, "Speculation and Experimentation in Early Poliomyelitis Research," *Clio Medica* 10 (1975): 1–22; Margaret L. Grimshaw, "Scientific Specialization and the Poliovirus Controversy in the Years before World War II," *Bulletin of the History of Medicine* 69, no. 1 (spring 1995): 44–65; Dorothy Horstmann, "The Poliomyelitis Story: A Scientific Hegira," *Yale Journal of Biology and Medicine* 58 (1985): 79–90; Thomas M. Rivers, "The Story of Research on Poliomyelitis," *Proceedings of the American Philosophical Society* 98, no. 4 (August 1954): 250–54; Frederick C. Robbins, "The History of Polio Vaccine Development," in *Vaccines*, ed. Stanley A. Plotkin and Walter

A. Orenstein (Philadelphia: Saunders, 1999), pp. 13–27. The standard history of medical research on poliomyelitis is Paul, *A History of Poliomyelitis.*

12. Simon Flexner, "The Contribution of Experimental to Human Poliomyelitis," *JAMA,* 55, no. 13 (September 24, 1910): 1111; Sidney D. Kramer, "Active Immunization against Poliomyelitis: A Comparative Study," part 1, "Attempts at Immunization of Monkeys and Children with Formalized Virus," *Journal of Immunology* 31, no. 3 (September 1936): 167.

13. I use the term "moratorium" to refer to both delays and suspensions in the human use of a medical innovation. Judith Swazey and Renée C. Fox, who coined the term, use it to refer to suspensions only. See "The Clinical Moratorium: A Case Study of Mitral Valve Surgery," in *Experimentation with Human Subjects,* ed. Paul A. Freund (New York: George Braziller, 1970), pp. 315–57.

14. Flexner, "The Contribution of Experimental to Human Poliomyelitis," p. 1111.

15. Ibid., pp. 1112–13.

16. Simon Flexner to Hans Zinsser, November 22, 1911, Flexner Papers, folder: Poliomyelitis (Zinsser, Hans).

17. Simon Flexner to Hans Zinsser, November 28, 1911, Flexner Papers, folder: Poliomyelitis (Zinsser, Hans).

18. Hans Zinsser to Simon Flexner, December 4, 1911, Flexner Papers, folder: Poliomyelitis (Zinsser, Hans).

19. Peter F. Olitsky and Herald R. Cox, "Experiments on Active Immunization against Experimental Poliomyelitis," *Journal of Experimental Medicine* 63 (1936): 109.

20. International Committee for the Study of Infantile Paralysis, *Poliomyelitis;* M. D. Stewart and C. P. Rhoads, "Intradermal versus Subcutaneous Immunization of Monkeys against Poliomyelitis," *Journal of Experimental Medicine* 49, no. 6 (June 1929): 959–73.

21. International Committee for the Study of Infantile Paralysis, *Poliomyelitis,* pp. 130–31. Because the risk of natural disease is higher during epidemics, the lesser-harm calculus is altered.

22. Kramer, "Active Immunization against Poliomyelitis, A Comparative Study," part 1, pp. 179–80. On Kramer's vaccine, see William H. Park, "The Prevention of Poliomyelitis," *New York State Journal of Medicine* 35, no. 16 (August 15, 1935): 819. Also see Frank L. Babbott Jr. to Robert A. Lambert (associate director, Rockefeller Foundation), January 9, 1935, and a four-page typescript beginning, "The plan for work as originally proposed . . ." [December 1934], RF Project Files, series 235a, box 4, folder 39: Long Island Medical College (Infantile Paralysis).

23. James P. Leake, "Poliomyelitis: Present Knowledge and Its Bearing on Control," *JAMA* 104, no. 14 (October 3, 1936): 1094–97.

24. For other accounts of the Park-Brodie and Kolmer vaccines, see Saul Benison, *Tom Rivers: Reflections on a Life in Medicine and Science* (Cambridge: MIT Press, 1967), pp. 184–90; Allan Chase, *Magic Shots* (New York: William Morrow, 1982), pp. 272–92; Lawrence B. Berk, "Polio Vaccine Trials of 1935," *Transactions of the College of Physicians of Philadelphia,* ser. 5, 11, no. 4 (1989): 321–336; Paul, *History of Poliomyelitis,* pp. 252–62; Susan E. Lederer, *Subjected to Science: Human Experimentation in America before the Second World War* (Baltimore: Johns Hopkins University Press, 1995), pp. 107–9.

25. Material on the ICM—originally called the Dermatological Research Laboratory (DRL)—and its role in producing Salvarsan include the thirty-eight-page typescript entitled "Research Institute of Cutaneous Medicine," DRL Records, box 3, folder: Research Institute of Cutaneous Medicine (Meeting Announcements and Miscellaneous Materials). Also see Jonathan Liebenau, *Medical Science and Medical Industry: The Formation of the American Pharmaceutical Industry* (Baltimore: Johns Hopkins University Press, 1987). Kolmer's early publications reported that his work was aided by a grant from the Daniel J. McCarthy Foundation Fund for Research in Neurology, Temple University. Kolmer produced his vaccine at the ICM. Later, he arranged for the William S. Merrill Company in Cincinnati to manufacture and distribute the immunizing agent. See John A. Kolmer, "Vaccination against Acute Anterior Poliomyelitis," *American Journal of Public Health* 26, no. 2 (February 1936): 126.

26. John F. Enders, Thomas H. Weller, and Frederick C. Robbins announced the development of tissue culture for poliovirus in "Cultivation of the Lansing Strain of Poliomyelitis Virus in Cultures of Various Human Embryonic Tissue," *Science* 109 (1949): 85–87. It was not until the 1960s that researchers became aware that polio vaccine grown in primate media could transmit simian viruses destructive to human health.

27. Numbers of animals tested from Paul, *History of Poliomyelitis*. The investigators' initial publications on animal trials were Maurice Brodie, "Active Immunization in Monkeys against Poliomyelitis with Germicidally Inactivated Virus, *Science* 79, no. 2061 (June 29, 1934): 594–95; and John A. Kolmer and Anna M. Rule, "Concerning Vaccination of Monkeys against Acute Anterior Poliomyelitis," *Journal of Immunology* 26, no. 6 (June 1934): 505–15.

28. Kolmer makes claims about the number of individuals receiving his vaccine in "Vaccination against Acute Anterior Poliomyelitis," and John A. Kolmer, "Active Immunization against Acute Anterior Poliomyelitis with Ricineolated Vaccine," *Journal of Immunology* 32, no. 5 (May 1937): 341–56. Other reports on the human testing of his immunizing agent include John A. Kolmer, George F. Klugh Jr., and Anna M. Rule, "A Successful Method for Vaccination against Acute Anterior Poliomyelitis," *JAMA* 104, no. 6 (February 9, 1935): 456–60; and John A. Kolmer, "Susceptibility and Immunity in Relation to Vaccination in Active Anterior Poliomyelitis," *JAMA* 105, no. 24 (December 14, 1935): 1956–62. On the number of individuals receiving Brodie's vaccine, see "Dr. Brodie Upholds Paralysis Vaccine: 10,000 Children Treated and None has Contracted the Disease, He Asserts," *New York Times*, November 3, 1935; copy in PBBC Records, box 2, Correspondence and Reports from Grantees, section 9 (New York University). Brodie and Park's accounts of the numbers receiving their immunizing agent were quite elastic. In an April 1935 letter to New York City's commissioner of hospitals, Park claimed that 15,000 children in California alone had been vaccinated (William H. Park to S. S. Goldwater, Commissioner's Files, 1935–37, box 28375, folder: Poliomyelitis). Brodie's publications on human testing include Brodie, "Active Immunization in Monkeys against Poliomyelitis with Germicidally Inactivated Virus," pp. 594–95; Maurice Brodie and William H. Park, "Active Immunization against Poliomyelitis," *JAMA* 105, no. 14 (October 5, 1935): 1089–93; Maurice Brodie and William H. Park, "Active Immunization against Poliomyelitis," *New York State Journal of Medicine* 35, no. 16 (August 15, 1935): 815–18; Maurice Brodie and William H. Park, "Active Immunization against Poliomyelitis," *American Journal of Public Health* 26, no. 2 (February 1936): 119–25.

29. Margaret Pittman, "The Regulation of Biologic Products, 1902–1972," in *National*

Institute of Allergy and Infectious Disease: Intramural Contributions, 1887–1987, ed. Harriet R. Greenwald and Victoria A. Harden (Washington, D.C.: National Institutes of Health, 1987), pp. 61–70; Paul D. Parkman and M. Carolyn Hardegree, "Regulation and the Testing of Vaccines," in *Vaccines*, ed. Stanley A. Plotkin and Walter A. Orenstein (Philadelphia: Saunders, 1999), pp. 1131–43.

30. Paul, *History of Poliomyelitis*, p. 255.

31. On methods for testing for polio antibodies, see Brodie and Park, "Active Immunization against Poliomyelitis," *JAMA*.

32. Park reported that, before vaccinating the six volunteers at the Department of Health Laboratories, he and Brodie tested the volunteers' blood for polio antibodies. After the vaccinations, blood from three was again tested, showing "the vaccine had given an increase in the amount of antibody." However, "no further tests were carried out because of the shortage of animals." See William H. Park to Jeremiah Milbank, November 28, 1934, PBBC Records, box 2, Correspondence and Reports from Grantees, section 9 (New York University); see also "Monkeys Lacking in Paralysis Test" (August 21, 1934), *PEB* Clipping Collection, folder: Kolmer, John.

33. Flexner's retirement is discussed in George W. Corner, *A History of the Rockefeller Institute* (New York: Rockefeller Institute Press, 1964), p. 324. On changes in the contemporary polio-research community, see Benison, "Speculation and Experimentation in Early Poliomyelitis Research," and Grimshaw, "Scientific Specialization and the Poliovirus Controversy."

34. Some members of the research community viewed this use of the news media as improper. In a note to Peyton Rous, Flexner remarked caustically that Park and Brodie's results had been "announced (sic!) in the daily press" (Simon Flexner to Peyton Rous, March 22, 1935, Flexner Papers, folder: Rous, Peyton, no. 9). This was not the first time that Park had used the press to generate demand for immunization. In 1895, a campaign in the press helped the New York City Public Health Department persuade the public to seek diphtheria antitoxin. See Evelynn M. Hammonds, *Childhood's Deadly Scourge: The Campaign to Control Diphtheria in New York City, 1880–1930* (Baltimore: Johns Hopkins University Press, 1999). Newspaper coverage of Kolmer's press releases included the following declaration: "Dr. John Kolmer announced today that vaccination of 22 children with the anti–infantile paralysis vaccine he developed has thus far met with entire success" (from "Paralysis Serum Given 22 Children," *Philadelphia Evening Bulletin*, September 5, 1934, *PEB* Clipping Collection, folder: Kolmer, John). The health commissioner of New York City issued an official press release about human inoculations of Brodie's vaccine on September 9, 1934 (PHS Records, box 60, folder: Poliomyelitis). Media coverage of the two vaccines began several months before this. The *PEB* Clipping Collection contains numerous articles on the two vaccines from the summer of 1934. Clippings on Brodie's vaccine from July include "Doctors Take Vaccine," *Philadelphia Evening Bulletin*, July 6, 1934 (folder: Park, William); "Doctors Take 2nd Dose of Paralysis Vaccine," *New York Herald Tribune*, July 11, 1934 (folder: Brodie, Maurice); and "Latest Serum May be Tested on 12 Orphans," *New York American*, July 9, 1934 (folder: Brodie, Maurice). Clippings on Kolmer's vaccine from August include "Infant Paralysis Serum Developed," *Philadelphia Evening Bulletin*, August 17, 1934; "Paralysis Vaccine Available Soon," *Philadelphia Evening Bulletin*, August 18, 1934; "Infant Paralysis Vaccine Reported: Serum Said to Immunize Children," *New York Times*, August 18, 1934; "Will Test Vaccine on 20 Children," *Philadelphia Evening Bulletin*, August 20, 1934;

and "Will Test Vaccine on Own Children," *Philadelphia Evening Bulletin,* August 21, 1934 (folder: Kolmer, John).

35. Brodie discussed early human tests with his vaccine at the New York Academy of Medicine on November 21, 1934. That month saw publication of his paper "Active Immunization of Children against Poliomyelitis with Formalin Inactivated Virus Suspension," *Proceedings of the Society for Experimental Biology and Medicine* 32, no. 2 (November 1934): 300–302. Kolmer's initial published account of human trials had appeared the previous month: "A Successful Method for Vaccination against Acute Anterior Poliomyelitis: Preliminary Report," *American Journal of Medical Science* 188 (October 1934): 510–14.

36. John Kolmer to Simon Flexner, December 27, 1932, Flexner Papers, folder: Kolmer, John.

37. "As you will find in reading River's book, the killed viruses do not give active immunity. They behave in an entirely different way from bacteria. If you have never worked with viruses, I wonder, would you not do better to study first the herpes virus infection in rabbits, rather than the more difficult experimental poliomyelitis in monkeys" (Simon Flexner to John Kolmer, January 10, 1933, Flexner Papers, folder: Kolmer, John).

38. Paul de Kruif to Jeremiah Milbank, April 3, 1935, PBBC Records, box 2, Correspondence and Reports from Grantees, section 9 (New York University). I found no records indicating whether Kolmer had requested PBBC funding.

39. Thomas Rivers to R. A. Lambert, January 7, 1935, RF Project Files, series 235a, box 4, folder 39: Long Island Medical College (Infantile Paralysis).

40. Simon Flexner to Peyton Rous, March 22, 1935, Flexner Papers, folder: Rous, Peyton, no. 9. Flexner consulted Peter Olitsky about Brodie's paper.

41. Thomas Rivers elaborating on Flexner's objections in "Discussion of Papers by William H. Park and Maurice Brodie and by John A. Kolmer on Poliomyelitis," Rivers Papers, folder: Discussion of Papers on Poliomyelitis, 1935. Rivers delivered this paper at the American Public Health Association meetings in Milwaukee, October 8, 1935. It is reprinted in Benison, *Tom Rivers,* pp. 599–601.

42. Simon Flexner to Peyton Rous, March 22, 1935, Flexner Papers, folder: Rous, Peyton, no. 9; Simon Flexner to Maurice Brodie, March 22, 1935, Flexner Papers, folder: Brodie, Maurice. I found no records indicating whether such a meeting took place.

43. "I believe it to be of urgent importance that you suggest to Park that he, Brodie, Charles Armstrong, and McCoy go into a huddle very soon—with the object of ironing out such discrepancies. As Armstrong stays, an hour's conversation between him and Brodie might explain everything that Brodie has left out of his published results." De Kruif was describing the outcome of a meeting with "McCoy and his men" taking place in late March 1935 (Paul de Kruif to Jeremiah Milbank, April 3, 1935, PBBC Records, box 2, Correspondence and Reports from Grantees, section 9 [New York University]).

44. De Kruif summarizes McCoy's position on Brodie's vaccine: "McCoy believes that, of all work now being done on the subject of immunization and prevention of poliomyelitis, that of Park and Brodie is the work that chiefly merits our support. He believes that even at this early date—i.e. before the President has turned over the money to us—we are justified in following Park's request for commitment of money, both for the laboratory as we've already done, and also for monkeys—a considerable number of which should be on hand within six weeks if anything is to be done this summer. . . . McCoy admits that he

hasn't much hope that the Brodie vaccine will be the answer to the prevention of poliomyelitis. But McCoy—as I told our Commission the evening of January 5—is the most skeptical man in the world" (Paul de Kruif to Jeremiah Milbank, April 3, 1935, PBBC Records, box 2, Correspondence and Reports from Grantees, section 9 (New York University).

45. "Dr. Morris Fishbein, secretary of the American Medical Association, said the Association had 'only the highest praise for Dr. Kolmer's work' but remarked that the vaccine is still in the experimental stages" (from "Will Test Vaccine on 20 Children," *Philadelphia Evening Bulletin*, August 20, 1934). Another article quotes Fishbein as saying: "Some doubt still exists as to the amount of free toxins available for use in preparations of the vaccine" (from "Doctor Praises Kolmer Vaccine," August 20, 1934). The "remarkable progress" comment is from this piece. Both articles found at the *PEB* Clipping Collection, folder: Kolmer, John.

46. "Hundreds Volunteer for Paralysis Serum," *Philadelphia Evening Bulletin*, July 7, 1934, Temple University Urban Archive, *PEB* Clipping Collection, folder: Kolmer, John. Flexner commented on popular demand for the polio vaccines: "The public is not only willing but eager to accept any treatment, preventive or curative, however experimental its scientific basis may be" ("Vaccination against Poliomyelitis," *Health News* 12, no. 34 [August 26, 1935]: 133). Also reported in "Poliomyelitis: Dr Flexner on the Present Status of Immunization by Serum," *New York Sun*, August 28, 1935, PBBC Records, box 2, Correspondence and Reports from Grantees, section 9 (New York University).

47. "Anti-Paralysis Serum Reported a Success in Wholesale Tests Made in California," *New York Times*, February 3, 1935, p. 21. Bert Hansen reports evidence of both widespread press coverage and intense public interest in laboratory-generated medical innovations beginning in the 1880s. See "New Images of a New Medicine: Visual Evidence for the Widespread Popularity of Therapeutic Discoveries in America after 1885," *Bulletin of the History of Medicine* 73, no. 4 (winter 1999): 629–78.

48. The statement includes the following sentence, which is crossed out by hand in the document: "With rabies (hydrophobia) for example, the chance of getting a paralysis from the inoculation of nerve tissue is enough for us to advise against the treatment unless the danger from the disease is real, and in this procedure paralysis results from only one in several thousand treatments, on the average" ("Inoculation against Poliomyelitis" [one-page typescript, dated February 22, 1935, with "H.S. Cummings, Surgeon General" typed at the bottom], NIH Records, 1930–48, General Files 0425P, box 15, folder: Misc Matters–Polio).

49. G. W. McCoy to L. L. Lumsden, August 23, 1935, NIH Records, 1930–48, General Files 0425P, box 15, folder: Polio (General).

50. On McCoy's official stances on such matters see Victor H. Kramer, *The National Institute of Health: A Study in Public Administration* (New Haven: Quinnipiack, 1937); Harry M. Marks, *The Progress of Experiment: Science and Therapeutic Reform in the United States, 1900–1990* (New York: Cambridge University Press, 1997), p. 74.

51. Rivers comments on Flexner's oversight of Olitsky's work in a letter to G. Foard McGinnes, July 1, 1935, Flexner Papers, folder: Rivers, Thomas, no. 4.

52. Thomas Rivers to G. Foard McGinnes, July 1, 1935, Flexner Papers, folder: Rivers, Thomas, no. 4. Schultz presented findings at the American Association of Pathologists and Bacteriologists in April. See E. W. Schultz and L. P. Gebhardt, "On the Problem of Immu-

nization against Poliomyelitis," *California and Western Medicine* 43, no. 2 (August 1935): 111–12. Olitsky and Cox would submit their results in October (Olitsky and Cox, "Experiments on Active Immunization against Experimental Poliomyelitis," pp. 109–25).

53. Memo by R. A. Lambert, dated July 2, 1935, reporting conversation with Kramer, RF Project Files, series 235A, box 4, folder 39: Long Island Medical College (Infantile Paralysis). Park wanted the publication of Kramer's results delayed.

54. Thomas Rivers to G. Foard McGinnes, July 1, 1935, Flexner Papers, folder: Rivers, Thomas, no. 4.

55. Thomas Rivers to G. Foard McGinnes, July 1, 1935, Flexner Papers, folder: Rivers, Thomas, no. 4.

56. A. G. Gilliam and R. H. Onstott, "Results of Field Studies with Poliomyelitis Vaccine," *American Journal of Public Health* 26, no. 2 (1936): 113.

57. W. Lloyd Aycock and C. C. Hudson, "The Development of Neutralizing Substances for Poliomyelitis Virus in Vaccinated and Unvaccinated Individuals, *New England Journal of Medicine* 214, no. 15 (1936): 715–18.

58. As De Kruif put it: "The attack rate of the disease is so low, that very large numbers of children must be vaccinated, and compared with non-vaccinated controls, in order to obtain figures that will be scientifically significant" ("Memorandum for the Information of the Members of the President's Birthday Ball Commission for Infantile Paralysis Research," [October 18, 1935], PBBC Records, box 2, Correspondence and Reports from Grantees, section 9 [New York University]). For comments on the disparity between notions about how best to conduct clinical trials and resources available for their conduct, see Harry M. Marks, "Notes from the Underground: The Social Organization of Therapeutic Research," in *Grand Rounds: One Hundred Years of Internal Medicine*, ed. Russell C. Maulitz and Diana E. Long (Philadelphia: University of Pennsylvania Press, 1988), pp. 297–336.

59. Memorandum from George W. McCoy to Assistant Surgeon General L. R. Thompson, dated August 28, 1935, PHS Records, General Files, 1924–35, box 60, folder: Poliomyelitis 0425. On risks associated with nerve tissue in rabies vaccines, see note 48 above.

60. De Kruif reported that, at a June 1935 medical advisory committee meeting, McCoy said, "Any vaccine, composed as Brodie's was, of tissue foreign to that of the human being (namely, monkey tissue) might, when given to many thousands of children, result in a certain number of dangerous, and even deadly reactions" (Paul de Kruif to Jeremiah Milbank, December 28, 1935, PBBC Records, box 2, Correspondence and Reports from Grantees, section 9 [New York University]). A copy of this letter is included in the typescript "Report on the Brodie Vaccine, 1934–35, Prepared by the Historical Division, April 21, 1954," NFIP Records, series: Procedures, folder: Vaccine, Polio, Brodie.

61. Kessel continues: "In each instance there was marked soreness at the point of injection and about 4 hours after the injection a generalized reaction with chills and fever developed, which lasted from 6 to 10 hours and then subsided" (John F. Kessel, "Discussion of Poliomyelitis Papers," *American Journal of Public Health* 26, no. 2 [February 1936]: 147).

62. "General reactions follow[ing] the vaccine were observed in 17 children (3.7 per cent) and in 4 were, at times, very disturbing" (Gilliam and Onstott, "Results of Field Studies with Poliomyelitis Vaccine," p. 116).

63. George W. McCoy to William H. Park, September 12, 1935, NIH Records, 1930–48, General Files 0425P, box 15, folder: Misc Matters–Polio.

64. Brodie's notarized report can be found in Rivers Papers, folder: Brodie, Maurice. The vaccinations had taken place during July, August, and September. The report of the cases of post-vaccination poliomyelitis is included in Rivers Papers, folders: Slemons, C. C., and Roehm, H. Kolmer's acknowledgment of poliomyelitis cases and deaths can be found in "Vaccination against Acute Anterior Poliomyelitis.

65. Simon Flexner to Thomas Rivers, October 5, 1935, Flexner Papers, folder: Rivers, Thomas, no. 4. Newspaper coverage of Flexner's *Science* article includes "Flexner Rejects Paralysis Vaccine," *New York Times*, November 1, 1935; "Paralysis Virus Held Unstable by Dr. Flexner," *New York Herald-Tribune*, November 1, 1935; "Dr. Brodie Upholds Paralysis Vaccine," *New York Times*, November 3, 1935. Copies of each of these articles can be found in PBBC Records, box 2, Correspondence and Reports from Grantees, section 9 (New York University).

66. Benison, *Tom Rivers*, p. 188.

67. "Discussion of Papers by William H. Park and Maurice Brodie and by John A. Kolmer on Poliomyelitis," Rivers Papers, folder: Discussion of Papers on Poliomyelitis, 1935; reprinted in Benison, *Tom Rivers*, pp. 599–601.

68. "Kolmer Defends Use of Vaccine," *Philadelphia Evening Bulletin*, October 9, 1935; "Dr. Kolmer is Sure Vaccine Is Safe," *Philadelphia Evening Bulletin*, October 10, 1935, *PEB* Clipping Collection, folder: Kolmer, John.

69. From a cover letter accompanying a legal brief submitted by A. Willcox to Herman Oliphant, general counsel of the Treasury Department: "I do not think that [Dr. Kolmer] has violated the law, or by the attached letter threatens to violate it. . . . There is no threat of violation unless we can say that a delivery of vaccine pursuant to the letter would constitute a 'sale, barter, or exchange.' As he expressly states there is no charge for the vaccine, I do not think there is a sale. . . . Dr. Leake would prefer to withdraw the request for opinion unless you feel you can rule favorably [that a violation of law has occurred]. . . . May I advise Dr. Leake that any opinion would have to be unfavorable?" Oliphant's response: "You may" (Treasury Department, interoffice communication from Mr. Willcox to Mr. Oliphant, October 23, 1935, with response from Mr. Oliphant, NIH Records, 1930–48, General Files 0425P, box 15, folder: Misc Matters–Polio).

70. Benison, *Tom Rivers*, p. 189. Leake's published comments are a great deal milder: "In any individual case the possibility should be left open that natural infection was operative, but the meaning of the series as a whole is clear to me, and I beg you (Dr. Kolmer) to desist from the human use of this vaccine" (James P. Leake, "Discussion of Poliomyelitis Papers," *American Journal of Public Health* 26, no. 2 [February, 1936]: 148). Benison noted the discrepancy between Leake's published remarks and Rivers's recollection and asked Leake what he had actually said. Leake reported that he did not remember his exact words but that he did recall using very harsh language (Bension, *Tom Rivers*, p. 190 n. 26).

71. "It appears that some question has arisen as to whether the officers of the Public Health Service might be liable in a libel action as a result of the publication of this statement. I am of the opinion that the statement is clearly not libelous" (Herman Oliphant, general counsel, to Josephine Roche, assistant secretary of the treasury, November 21,

1935, NIH Records, 1930–48, General Files, classification 0425P, box 15, folder: Misc Matters–Polio).

72. James P. Leake, "Poliomyelitis Following Vaccination against the Disease," *JAMA* 105, no. 26 (December 28, 1935): 2152.

73. A copy of Leake's original draft is found with Oliphant's memo: Herman Oliphant to Josephine Roche, November 21, 1935, NIH Records, 1930–48, General Files 0425P, box 15, folder: Misc Matters–Polio.

74. Discussion of the first case of polio subsequent to immunization with the Brodie vaccine is found in an undated typescript titled "From Health Commissioner John L. Rice," Commissioner's Files, 1935–37, box 28375, folder: Poliomyelitis. Also see "Paralysis Virus Held Unstable by Dr. Flexner . . . Dr. Park Differs, Telling of Results on 9,000 Cases," *New York Herald-Tribune*, November 1, 1935; copy found in PBBC Records, box 2, Correspondence and Reports from Grantees, section 9 (New York University). Park insisted that all modified preparations were tested for safety with monkeys before human use (William H. Park to Paul de Kruif, December 19, 1935, NIH Records, 1930–48, General Files 0425P, box 15, folder: Misc Matters–Polio).

75. "In the opinion of those whom I consulted as well as in my own judgement, the reasonableness is nearly absolute that these infections [two cases of poliomyelitis] were induced by the vaccinations" (Karl F. Meyer to Joseph K. Smith, December 13, 1935, Bancroft Library, Karl F. Meyer Papers, carton 94, folder 7: Brodie Vaccine, 1935–36). After receiving a written account of Meyer's assessment, Leake wrote to Meyer: "It was good to see your signature. I am enclosing a statement not yet published and at present confidential. It has been mimeographed so that it may be sent to the various persons who have supplied the information; you can see the delicate situation of the physicians and parents. Until the recent word from California, I was somewhat in doubt about the safety of the Brodie vaccine" (James P. Leake to Karl F. Meyer, December 14, 1935, Meyer Papers, carton 94, folder 7: Brodie Vaccine, 1935–36).

76. "Status of Vaccination against Poliomyelitis," *JAMA* 107, no. 9 (August 29, 1936): 717. Objections by California physicians included the following: "It does not appear as if the evidence at present at hand is sufficient to prove either danger or effectiveness of the vaccine" (Emil Bogen to Maurice Brodie, December 30, 1935). Park wrote to Greer at the PBBC on February 26, 1936, saying that health officers in Kern County felt "that there is very little chance that the vaccine led to any of the cases there" and they were "anxious to go on with the vaccination." Both letters can be found in PBBC Records, box 2, Correspondence and Reports from Grantees, section 9 (New York University).

77. "McCoy and Leake felt that the couple of children vaccinated, who had come down with poliomyelitis at a time suspiciously close to vaccination, *might* have been infected with the disease by the vaccine itself. McCoy said that this was not amenable to proof, but that it looked suspicious. These suspicions are strengthened, but again not proved, by the fact that Brodie had been found to be exposing the infected monkey tissue to formaldehyde for shorter and shorter times" (Paul de Kruif to Jeremiah Milbank, December 28, 1935, PBBC Records, box 2, Correspondence and Reports from Grantees, section 9 [New York University]; emphasis in the original).

78. I found no records indicating whether lawsuits were initiated in response to the incidents of post-vaccination polio in 1935.

79. Paul de Kruif to Jeremiah Milbank, December 28, 1935, PBBC Records, box 2, Correspondence and Reports from Grantees, section 9 (New York University).

80. William H. Park to Paul de Kruif, December 19, 1935, NIH Records, 1930–48, General Files 9425P, box 15, folder: Misc Matters–Polio.

81. William H. Park to George W. McCoy, December 4, 1935, NIH Records, 1930–48, General Files 0425P, box 15, folder: Misc Matters–Polio.

82. Jeremiah Milbank to George W. McCoy, December 31, 1935, PBBC Records, box 2, Correspondence and Reports from Grantees, section 9 (New York University). Park had written to de Kruif about the impact Leake's article had had on the PBBC advisory board: "It seems to me that Dr. Leake may have involuntarily influenced the committee by putting the Kolmer deaths and cases on the same sheet before the Brodie cases so that the horror of the committee over the several fatalities with the Kolmer vaccine carried through" (William H. Park to Paul de Kruif, December 19, 1935, NIH Records, 1930–48, General Files 0425P, box 15, folder: Misc Matters–Polio).

83. Karl F. Meyer to Joseph K. Smith, December 13, 1935, Meyer Papers, carton 94, folder 7: Brodie Vaccine, 1935–36. With access to lot numbers, researchers would have been able to figure out how long the poliovirus given to afflicted recipients had been treated with formalin.

84. Karl F. Meyer to Joseph K. Smith, December 13, 1935, Meyer Papers, carton 94, folder 7: Brodie Vaccine, 1935–36. Meyer's rebuke was not entirely fair. In a letter to Park written six months earlier, Smith had made it clear that the Kern County Health Department had insufficient resources to keep track of research data: "The only condition under which we could carry out the selection of an equal number of controls per number of persons vaccinated in Kern County is that the National Institutes of Health send us trained persons to actually do the work of this part of the vaccination program. . . . We must let you know that our staff is taxed to the limit with the present emergency and have no time for additional work of selecting controls and keeping data beyond what has already been kept" (Joseph K. Smith, Kern County health officer, to William H. Park, [July 1935]). The NIH decided against pursuing the collection of control-group data in Kern County because the incidence of polio there was already high (James P. Leake to William. H. Park, July 30, 1935). Both the Smith and the Leake letters can be found in the NIH Records, 1930–48, General Files 0425P, box 15, folder: Poliomyelitis in North Carolina, 1935 (Drs. Leake and Alex Gilliam).

85. PHS Records, General Files, box 60, folder: Poliomyelitis. In September 1934, the New York City health commissioner, John L. Rice, received letters of protest about the use of orphans in the testing of polio vaccines. See Commissioner's Files 1934, box 25957, folder: Poliomyelitis.

86. Benison, *Tom Rivers,* p. 189.

87. Paul de Kruif to Jeremiah Milbank, December 28, 1935, PBBC Records, box 2, Correspondence and Reports from Grantees, section 9 (New York University).

88. Paul, *History of Poliomyelitis,* pp. 261–62.

89. On the atheoretical character of early vaccine research, see Anne Marie Moulin, "La Métaphore vaccine: De l'inoculation à la vaccinologie," *History and Philosophy of Life Science* 14 (1992): 271–97.

90. In December 1935, newspapers reported the vaccine-related deaths, Leake's article

in *JAMA,* and the PBBC's decision to stop use of the Park-Brodie vaccine. See clippings at PBBC Records, box 2, Correspondence and Reports from Grantees, section 9 (New York University).

Chapter Three

1. Some of these organizations both employed scientists and provided research support. Others provided external research funding only.

2. Before the start of their PBBC funding, Brodie and Park wrote that their research "was aided by grants from the Rockefeller and New York Foundations and from Mr. Jeremiah Milbank" (Maurice Brodie and William H. Park, "Active Immunization against Poliomyelitis," *JAMA* 105, no. 14 [October 5, 1935]: 1089). Milbank was a major contributor to the PBBC and provided interim funding to Park before the commission issued its award. On PBBC support for Park and Brodie, see PBBC Records, box 2, Correspondence and Reports from Grantees, section 9 (New York University). On Rockefeller Foundation support, see RF Project Files, series 235a, box 4, folder 41: NYC Laboratories (Poliomyelitis). On New York Foundation funding, see NYF Records, folder: New York University (Poliomyelitis Fund).

3. Kolmer reported that his work was "aided by grants from the Daniel J. McCarthy Foundation Fund for Research on Neurology of Temple University and two anonymous donations" (John A. Kolmer, George F. Klugh Jr., and Anna M. Rule, "A Successful Method for Vaccination against Acute Anterior Poliomyelitis," *JAMA* 104, no. 6 [February 9, 1935]: 456). He mentions his arrangement with the pharmaceutical firm William S. Merrill Company in John A. Kolmer, "Vaccination against Acute Anterior Poliomyelitis," *American Journal of Public Health* 26, no. 2 (February 1936): 128.

4. See the discussion of George McCoy's objections in chapter 2.

5. The Park-Brodie project records at the New York Foundation and Rockefeller Foundation contain no discussion of the safety of their polio vaccine nor—apart from their own comments in routine project summaries—any discussion of procedures used during human testing.

6. Available records provide no information on dynamics internal to the ICM concerning Kolmer's polio vaccine. The College of Physicians of Philadelphia holds a small collection of documents from the ICM, but apart from lists of publications by institute researchers, these holdings include no mention of Kolmer's polio-vaccine development and testing.

7. Descriptions of Kramer's vaccine can be found in RF Project Files, series 235A, box 4, folder 39: Long Island Medical School, Infantile Paralysis. See Frank L. Babbott Jr., Long Island College of Medicine, to Robert A. Lambert, associate director of the Rockefeller Foundation, January 9, 1935. Also see a four-page typescript beginning, "The plan of work as originally proposed . . . " [December 1934]. Additional comments are found in William H. Park, "The Prevention of Poliomyelitis," *New York State Journal of Medicine* 35, no. 1 (August 15, 1935): 819; and T. E. Boyd, "Immunization against Poliomyelitis," *Bacteriological Review* 17, supplement (December 1953): 425–26.

8. On Flexner's work on poliomyelitis in the early 1930s, see "Immunity to Human and Passage Poliomyelitis Virus," *Transactions of the Association of American Physicians* 47 (1932): 109–115, and "Experiments on Active Poliomyelitis" (report on the Proceedings of the Association of American Physicians, May 1932) *JAMA* 99, no. 1 (July 2, 1932): 69–70.

9. As mentioned in chapter 2, it was Kramer who noted, in the aftermath of the Kolmer and Park-Brodie trials, that the incidence of polio was low and that, for human use of a vaccine to be justified, risks of the immunizing agent needed to be lower than the hazards of the natural disease. See Sidney D. Kramer, "Active Immunization against Poliomyelitis: A Comparative Study," part 1, "Attempts at Immunization of Monkeys and Children with Formalized Virus," *Journal of Immunology* 31, no. 3 (September 1936): 167–81.

10. "Paralysis Serum Not for Babies Yet," *New York Times* clipping, dated April 27, 1932, AV Papers, box 17, folder 12: Antivivisection Correspondence, "K." The *Times* article incorrectly lists Kramer's name as Dr. Hyman L. Kramer. Correspondence in the Rockefeller Antivivisection Papers makes it clear that the person being quoted was Sidney D. Kramer. Kramer's comment in the *New York Times* may have been triggered by contemporary scientific literature on Pasteur's rabies vaccine. In the late 1920s and early 1930s, researchers collected and published systematic evidence on the high morbidity and mortality associated with immunization against rabies (see above, chapter 1, note 43). The *Times* article includes no description of Kramer's immunizing agent. It may have been one referred to by Frank Babbott, who states that, when Kramer was at Harvard, he worked with Aycock on a vaccine initially developed by C. P. Rhoads—composed of poliovirus adsorbed in "aluminium hydroxide." See Frank L. Babbott Jr. to Robert A. Lambert, January 9, 1935, RF Project Files, series 235A, box 4, folder 39: Long Island Medical School, Infantile Paralysis.

11. Peyton Rous wrote to Kramer insisting that the younger researcher retract his statement because it appeared to substantiate the antivivisectionists' claim that investigators were conducting wholesale experimentation on children: "This year the anti-vivisectionists of New York State caused more trouble to the doctors defending freedom of animal research than in many past years. There is every indication that next year the trouble will be very serious. . . . At each hearing before the legislature the anti-vivisectionists bring forward, among their various claims, one of wholesale experimentation upon children which thus far we have been able to rebut. Now it would seem as if this claim had found substantiation in the assertion published in the New York Times. . . . The statement published in the Times will do great harm, indeed has already done it" (Peyton Rous to Sidney Kramer, May 3, 1932). Kramer responded in letter dated May 27: "The quotation attributed to me in the press is a stupid and flagrant misstatement and does not represent the opinion of either the Commission or myself personally." When pressed about what he did say, Kramer responded (in at letter to Rous dated June 11): "I told [the reporter] that before anything is to be used on human beings, great care must be taken to ascertain the safety of the procedure. I furthermore told him that we had, in a measure, more facilities available for testing various processes now than ever before and went on to say that such added precautions are now more available possibly, than in the days of Pasteur." The following handwritten note from Rous is attached to Kramer's letter: "Dear Dr. Flexner: This ends the Kramer episode, I should think. What wriggling! PR." And, on the bottom of Rous's note, in Simon Flexner's handwriting: "Thanks. Excellent. SF." Correspondence from the AV Papers, Record Group 600–1, box 17, folder 12: Antivivisection Correspondence, "K."

12. Kramer's Rockefeller Foundation project files are at RF Project Files, series 235A, box 4, folder 39: Long Island Medical School, Infantile Paralysis. Other materials that might shed light on Kramer's decision making are limited. The papers of the Harvard Infantile Paralysis Commission, where Kramer worked under Lloyd Aycock during the early

1930s, contain few entries from this period. Nor are there records at Long Island Medical College on Kramer's polio research.

13. Simon Flexner to Peyton Rous, March 22, 1935, Flexner Papers, folder: Rous, Peyton, no. 9.

14. Researchers typically view the first human trial of a vaccine as riskier than subsequent trials, assuming that the first experiment generated no human injuries. For this reason, Stokes's experiments would have been seen as less hazardous than Francis's trial. At the same time, the much greater size of Stokes's subject pool would have been seen as increasing the chance for a human accident associated with vaccine use.

15. Thomas Francis Jr., "Transmission of Influenza by a Filterable Virus," *Science* 80, no. 2081 (November 16, 1934): 457–59; Wilson Smith, C. H. Andrews, and P. P. Laidlaw, "A Virus Obtained from Influenza Patients," *Lancet*, July 8, 1933, pp. 66–68.

16. Preparation of the vaccine is described in Thomas Francis Jr., "Cultivation of Human Influenza Virus in an Artificial Medium," *Science* 82, no. 2128 (1935): 353–54. Homer F. Swift, of the Rockefeller Institute Hospital, discussed reasons for considering Francis's virus attenuated: "The passage of a virus through animals belonging to another species causes that virus to become attenuated in respect to the original species. It can then be used as an immunizing agent for the first species. Dr. Francis has been able to pass the influenza virus through many generations of mice, and thus hopes that it has lost much of its virulence for man. Still another way to attenuate viruses is by repeated cultivation in vitro. During the past few months Dr. Francis and Dr. Magill have been able to cultivate influenza virus and hope to show that this is a good immunizing agent" (Homer F. Swift to Charles R. Stockard, August 29, 1935, Business Manager's Files, box 14, folder: Influenza, 1918–45).

17. Francis reported on the outcome of his first human trial in Thomas Francis Jr. and T. P. Magill, "Vaccination of Human Subjects with Virus of Human Influenza," *Proceedings of the Society for Experimental Biology and Medicine* 33, no. 4 (January, 1936): 604–6. He discusses the second in Thomas Francis Jr. and T. P. Magill, "The Antibody Response of Human Subjects Vaccinated with the Virus of Human Influenza," *Journal of Experimental Medicine* 65, no. 2 (1937): 251–59.

18. "In September and October of 1935, several members of the hospital staff and a few hospitalized children who showed only small amounts of neutralizing substances in their sera against the human and swine flu viruses . . . were injected intramuscularly with both agents in an active state" (Joseph Stokes Jr. et al., "Results of Immunization by Means of Active Virus of Human Influenza," *Journal of Clinical Investigation* 16, no. 2 (1937): 237–38.

19. Ibid., pp. 237–43; Joseph Stokes Jr., Aims C. McGuinness, Paul H. Langer, and Dorothy Shaw, "Vaccination against Epidemic Influenza with Active Virus of Human Influenza," *American Journal of Medical Sciences* 94 (1937): 757–68.

20. Of the $2,100, $1,500 went toward expenses of isolating subjects at the Rockefeller Institute Hospital and $600 toward honoraria for subjects—most of whom received a sum of $50. See [Edric B. Smith], Rockefeller Institute business manager, to Rufus Cole, director of the Rockefeller Hospital, September 6, 1935, Business Manager's Files, box 14, folder: Influenza, 1918–45. Francis appears to have conducted the second set of human inoculations under the auspices of the Rockefeller Foundation. The publication discussing Fran-

cis's expanded trial states that the research was from the Foundation's laboratories. See Thomas Francis Jr. and T. P. Magill, "The Antibody Response of Human Subjects Vaccinated with the Virus of Human Influenza," *Journal of Experimental Medicine* 65, no. 2 (1937): 251–59. Francis left the Rockefeller Institute in 1935. A thirteen-page typescript entitled "The Foundation's Research Center in New York," dated 1946, indicates that Francis worked at the IHD laboratories from 1936 to 1938 (RF Project Files, series 100, box 11, folder 92: International Health Division–Laboratories–History, 1942–50).

21. The Children's Hospital Influenza Fund (primarily donations from Abington Hospital) covered $70 in monthly salary support for Stokes's laboratory staff while the University of Pennsylvania covered $150 in monthly salary support. See the three-page typescript entitled "Influenza Study" (with handwritten comment, "sent to Dr. Gittings, 6/21/37"), Stokes Papers, box: Influenza no. 1, folder: Influenza Studies no. 3. Stokes describes this source as "some funds provided by two of the members of the Board at the Abington Memorial Hospital." See Joseph Stokes Jr. to John A. Ferrell at the Rockefeller Foundation, January 22, 1937, RF Project Files, series 241, box 4, folder 54: University of Pennsylvania (Influenza Studies), 1936–1938. A document in the Stokes Papers (circa 1936) indicates that, each month, Abington Hospital sent a gift of $250 to Stokes of which $190 was allocated to the "Children's Hospital Influenza Fund." See the one-page typescript "Influenza," Stokes Papers, box: Influenza no. 2, folder: Influenza no. 19 (Rockefeller Fund). Stokes solicited and received other charitable donations. A notice appeared in the *Readers Digest* (circa February 1936) announcing an effort to raise $25,000 for influenza research. This resulted in a number of contributions, including a check for $1,000 from an individual donor. See Roy Alan Van Clief to Children's Hospital of Philadelphia, February 21, 1936, Stokes Papers, box: Influenza no. 2, folder: Influenza no. 19 (Rockefeller Fund no. 1).

22. "Financial assistance to the amount of approximately $2,500 yearly has been granted toward this work by the Bureau of Animal Industries, United States Department of Agriculture, because of the relationship of the studies to swine influenza" (Joseph Stokes Jr. to Dr. Augustus Knight, May 21, 1938, Stokes Papers, box: Influenza no. 3, folder: Influenza Study no. 10). A memo dated January 29, 1936, describes a meeting about collaborative research on swine flu attended by Stokes, several University of Pennsylvania Veterinary School faculty, and a representative of Sharp & Dohme (Stokes Papers, box: Influenza no. 3, folder: Influenza no. 50).

23. Documentation on Rockefeller Foundation support for Stokes's influenza research is found in RF Project Files, series 241, box 4, folder 53: University of Pennsylvania (Influenza Studies), 1936–38. Also see "Influenza Study," Stokes Papers, box: Influenza no. 1, folder: Influenza Studies no. 3.

24. Homer F. Swift to Charles R. Stockard, August 29, 1935, Business Manager's Files, box 14, folder: Influenza, 1918–45. Stockard was a member of the Rockefeller Institute Board of Scientific Directors. George G. Corner discusses Institute policy on experiments with patients in *History of the Rockefeller Institute* (New York: Rockefeller Institute Press, 1964), p. 97. Also see Susan E. Lederer, *Subjected to Science: Human Experimentation in America before the Second World War* (Baltimore: Johns Hopkins University Press, 1995), p. 84.

25. Homer F. Swift to Simon Flexner, September 8, 1935, Business Manager's Files, box 14, folder: Influenza, 1918–45. Others at the Rockefeller Institute also invoked risk-benefit formulations when making arguments about Francis's trial. On October 8, 1935,

Rufus Cole wrote to Herbert Gasser, who had just succeeded Flexner as the Institute's scientific director. At issue was whether subjects for Francis's second trial should be restricted to physicians and medical students: "Mr. Debevoise [the Institute's lawyer] felt that, if possible, we should use medical students or doctors only, but he now realizes that that may be impossible, and, in view of the great importance of the work, he thinks we are justified in taking chances" (Business Manager's Files, box 14, folder: Influenza, 1918–45).

26. Drafts of the consent form are found in Business Manager's Files, box 14, folder: Influenza, 1918–45. On the recruitment of Francis's subjects, who were medical students at New York University, see "Report of Dr. Francis (assisted by Dr. Magill)," p. 168, Reports to RIMR Scientific Directors, box 6, volume 24, 1935–36, pp. 168–70.

27. "Dr. Cole's general approval is not altogether convincing to me since he wants the work held off until his return" (R. C. Stockard to Edric B. Smith, August 16, 1935, Business Manager's Files, box 14, folder: Influenza, 1918–45).

28. In a letter dated August 26, 1935, Homer Swift directed Francis away from nasal exposure and toward use of injections: "Of course I realize that the final test of their immunity would be the nasal inoculation; but might it not be possible to see whether people immunized in this way [via injection] would have a fair degree of protective antibodies develop in their serum? If this were true it would be fair presumptive evidence that they were immune. It may be that Mudd [at the University of Pennsylvania] or someone else will inoculate volunteers with the living virus and show that it is infective for man. If this happens you will be spared this part of the work and can devote the main part of your physical facilities and energies to the problem of protective immunization" (Business Manager's Files, box 14, folder: Influenza, 1918–45). Francis's earlier correspondence makes it clear that he wanted to conduct an experiment inducing clinical symptoms of influenza in human subjects. On May 31, 1935, Francis wrote to Simon Flexner: "I should like to talk with you concerning the possibility of attempting to transfer influenza to human volunteers. At the moment I am somewhat undecided whether human infection or human immunization experiments are the more important. Personally, I lean toward the former" (Flexner Papers, folder: Francis, Thomas Jr., no. 1). By June, Francis was even clearer about his preference: "I am trying at the present time to get things lined up for an experiment for the infection of humans" (Thomas Francis to Rufus Cole, June 27, 1935, Francis Papers, box 1, folder: Co.).

29. I found no evidence of efforts by his sponsors to monitor Stokes's 1935–38 influenza trials in either Stokes's own papers or in his Rockefeller Foundation project files. The latter are located in RF Project Files, series 241, box 4, folder 53: University of Pennsylvania (Influenza Studies), 1936–38. Records on support from the Abington Hospital Fund are found in Stokes Papers, box: Influenza no. 19, folder: Rockefeller Fund 1. My search at the National Archives for holdings on U.S. Department of Agriculture funding for influenza studies at the University of Pennsylvania yielded no relevant material.

30. Seven-page typescript entitled "Influenza, Progress Report—May 15, 1936," Stokes Papers, box: Influenza no. 2, folder: Influenza no. 30.

31. These institutions included the State Colony in New Lisbon, the State Village for Epileptics at Skillman, the New Jersey State Home for Boys at Jamesburg (a correctional facility), the Vineland State Colony, and the Vineland Training School. See the five-page typescript entitled "Description of Studies," Stokes Papers, box: Influenza no. 2, folder: Influenza no. 23 (Rockefeller Fund 5).

32. Stokes was in frequent correspondence with officials managing the custodial facilities where he conducted influenza experiments. In his efforts to gain access, Stokes pointed to evidence suggesting the safety of human inoculations with live influenza virus. See, for example, his letter of November 16, 1935, to Dr. Ellen Potter, director of medicine of the State of New Jersey Department of Institutions and Agencies, Stokes Papers, box: Influenza no. 1, folder: Influenza Studies no. 6a.

33. "We are not interested in supporting at this stage of developments any plans for wide distribution of the virus for use by outside physicians as we feel that much additional experimental work will need to be done before we shall be safe in encouraging the general use of vaccines outside" (statement by W. A. Sawyer, director of the International Health Division, Rockefeller Foundation, interoffice correspondence, dated May 3, 1937, RF Project Files, series 241, box 4, folder 53: University of Pennsylvania [Influenza Studies], 1936–38).

34. Sabin, among others, argued vigorously against adoption of Salk's vaccine on the grounds that a killed-virus preparation would provide only short-lived immunity. See Marcia L. Meldrum, "The Historical Feud over Polio Vaccine: How Could a Killed Vaccine Contain a Natural Disease?" *Western Journal of Medicine* 171 (October 1999): 271–73. Most of the secondary sources on Salk's and Sabin's polio-vaccine research discuss controversy over the preferability of killed or live vaccines

35. This meeting, on immunization in poliomyelitis, was held in Hershey, Pennsylvania, March 15–17, 1951. See the typescript, dated March 1951, entitled "Proceedings of Round Table Conference on Immunization in Poliomyelitis," prepared by the National Foundation for Infantile Paralysis, pp. 155–60, NFIP Materials, Cincinnati Medical Heritage Center. On the reaction of polio researchers to Koprowski's announcement, see John R. Paul, *A History of Poliomyelitis* (New Haven: Yale University Press, 1971), p. 442.

36. John R. Paul conducted human tests of killed-virus preparations before 1950 but did not report this until later. Paul described these studies at a March 1955 meeting of the National Foundation Subcommittee on Live Virus Immunization. Henry Kumm, who became the Foundation's research director in September 1953, recounts Paul's discussion. "Dr. John Paul then proceeded to tell us about investigations now underway at the Southbury Training School, a Connecticut Mental Institution with approximately 1,000 patients. Studies were begun there in 1946 and killed virus was first fed to inmates in 1947 and 1948." The quotation is an excerpt from Kumm's diary entry for Monday, March 7, 1955, American Philosophical Society, Thomas Rivers Papers, folder: Kumm, Henry, no. 1.

37. Hilary Koprowski, "Immunization of Man against Poliomyelitis with Attenuated Preparation of Live Virus," *Annals of the New York Academy of Sciences* 61 (September 1955): 1039.

38. G. W. A. Dick et al., "Vaccination against Poliomyelitis with Live Virus Vaccines," part 2, "A Trial of SM Type I Attenuated Poliomyelitis Virus Vaccine," *British Medical Journal*, January 12, 1957, pp. 65–70; and G. W. A. Dick and D. S. Dane, "Vaccination against Poliomyelitis with Live Virus Vaccines," part 3, "The Evaluation of TN and SM Virus Vaccines" *British Medical Journal*, January 12, 1957, pp. 70–74.

39. Hilary Koprowski, George Jervis, and Thomas W. Norton, "Immune Response in Human Volunteers upon Oral Administration of a Rodent-Adapted Strain of Poliomyelitis Virus," *American Journal of Hygiene* 55, no. 1 (1952): 108–26.

40. On the live-polio vaccine trials conducted at Sonoma State (1953), Woodbine (1954), Sonoma State (1954–55) and Clinton Farms (1956), see, respectively, Hilary Koprowski et al., "Further Studies on Oral Administration of Living Poliomyelitis Virus to Human Subjects, *Proceedings of the Society of Experimental Biology and Medicine* 82 (February 1953): 277–80; Hilary Koprowski et al., "Immunization of Children by the Feeding of Living Attenuated Type I and Type II Poliomyelitis Virus and the Intramuscular Injection of Immune Serum Globulin," *American Journal of Medical Sciences* 232, no. 4 (October 1956): 378–88; Hilary Koprowski et al., "Clinical Investigations on Attenuated Strains of Poliomyelitis Virus," *JAMA* 160: 11 (March 17, 1956): 954–66; Hilary Koprowski et al., "Immunization of Infants with Living Attenuated Poliomyelitis Virus," *JAMA* 162, no. 14 (December 1, 1956): 1281–88. As T. E. Boyd noted, "much of the developmental work carried out at the Lederle Laboratories is unpublished." See the twenty-eight-page typescript, dated November 1958, entitled "Live-Virus Poliomyelitis Vaccines," NFIP Records, series: Procedures, folder: Vaccine, Polio, Sabin 1955.

41. Albert B. Sabin, "Immunization of Chimpanzees and Human Beings with Avirulent Strain of Poliomyelitis Virus," *Annals of the New York Academy of Medicine* 61, art. 4 (September 27, 1955): 1050–56; Albert B. Sabin, "Behavior of Chimpanzee-Avirulent Poliomyelitis Viruses in Experimentally Infected Human Volunteers," *American Journal of the Medical Sciences,* July 1955, pp. 1–8; Albert B. Sabin, "Present Status of Attenuated Live-Virus Poliomyelitis Vaccine," *JAMA* 162, no. 18 (December 29, 1956): 1589–96.

42. Hilary Koprowski, "Historical Aspects of the Development of Live Virus Vaccine in Poliomyelitis," *British Medical Journal,* July 9, 1960, p. 86. Koprowski's two collaborators were Thomas Norton, his assistant at Lederle, and George Jervis, a physician at Letchworth Village.

43. Koprowski's report of his first human trial at Letchworth Village refers to subjects as "volunteers" without elaborating how or from whom consent was obtained. Other of his publications state that consent was secured from subjects' parents. As noted earlier, it was often state health officials and managers of custodial facilities providing access to subjects who required consent and imposed measures to control risks. Before the 1954–55 polio-vaccine experiment at Sonoma State Hospital, Koprowski's research team meet with hospital physicians and California state health officers. A memo describing this meeting indicates that hospital administrators required that consent be obtained from subjects' parents or guardians. Hospital administrators also required that publicity about the trial be kept to a minimum. All participants concurred that vaccine recipients would be held in strict isolation during the study. In addition, state health officials made plans to secure advice from the Department of Public Health's legal counsel about the possibility that a lawsuit might arise in the event that a subject contracted polio. See the interoffice memorandum from Dr. Nelsen (medical director) to Dr. Porter (hospital superintendent), Sonoma State Hospital, May 5, 1954, Sabin Papers, drawer: Oral Polio Vaccine Production and Human Test, folder: Poliomyelitis, NFIP Correspondence, Human Tests. Sabin obtained the document from Karl Meyer, who attended the meeting.

44. The Foundation's Committee on Virus Research and Epidemiology discussed Sabin's proposed clinical trial at its meeting on April 5, 1954. Kumm wrote to Sabin that "the members of [that] committee . . . were not willing to recommend that you proceed with trials on human beings immediately. Instead it was decided to refer this question to the Vaccine Committee" (Henry Kumm to Albert Sabin, April 20, 1954, Sabin Papers,

drawer: Oral Polio Vaccine Production and Human Test, folder: Poliomyelitis NFIP Correspondence, Human Tests). On arrangements for Sabin to present his proposal to the Vaccine Advisory Committee, see Henry W. Kumm to Thomas Rivers, September 23, 1954,
Rivers Papers, folder: Kumm, Henry, no. 1. The meetings of another of the National Foundation scientific panels, referred to often as the Immunization Committee, included the
better part of the national colleague network of polio-vaccine researchers. Louis Galambos
and Jane Eliot Sewell write that vaccine development coordinated by the National Foundation involved a network of private and public institutions and was "cooperative technical research guided by a committee." See Louis Galambos and Jane Eliot Sewell, *Networks of Innovation: Vaccine Development at Merck, Sharp and Dohme, and Mulford, 1895–1995*
(Cambridge: Cambridge University Press, 1995), p. 59.

45. This subcommittee was composed of a handful of Foundation-funded researchers
who were actively testing live polio strains. By the mid-1950s, Koprowksi and Sabin were
not alone in conducting human trials with live viruses. In March 1955, Morris Schaeffer, at
the virus laboratory of the U.S. Public Health Service Communicable Disease Center in
Montgomery, was about to embark on a small trial of Type I polio strains at Pineview
Manor, an institution in Alabama for the mentally disabled. Also, John Paul and Joseph
Melnick at Yale were preparing to conduct a small trial of Type III virus strains at Southbury Training School in Connecticut. In 1957, Herald Cox began human tests of newly developed stains of live poliovirus. Cox took over Lederle Laboratories' polio-vaccine effort in
1957, when Koprowski left the company for a job at the Wistar Institute. On trials by
Schaeffer and by Melnick and Paul, see the nine-page typescript "Minutes of the Meeting of
the Subcommittee on Live Virus Immunization of the N.F.I.P. held at the Children's Hospital and Research Foundation in Cincinnati on 7–8 March 1955," Sabin Papers, box M20–
128, folder: Poliomyelitis NFIP, Live Virus Vaccine Committee. Henry Kumm, the National
Foundation's research director, attended this meeting, and a copy of his notes on the proceedings is found in the Rivers Papers, folder: Kumm, Henry, no. 1.

46. Henry Kumm to Albert Sabin, March 22, 1954. Sabin responded to Kumm's concerns in a letter of March 29, 1954. For both documents, see Sabin Papers, drawer: Oral Polio Vaccine Production and Human Test, folder: Poliomyelitis, NFIP Correspondence, Human Tests. A copy of the second letter can be found also in Rivers Papers, folder: Sabin,
Albert, no. 2.

47. "Dr. Rivers told me that the authorization which I now have from the NFIP for
studies on human volunteers applied only to the 3 strains with which I have worked thus
far, and the studies on new strains would have to be approved by the appropriated committee of the NFIP" (Albert Sabin to Henry Kumm, May 26, 1955, Sabin Papers, drawer: Oral
Polio Vaccine Production and Human Test, folder: Poliomyelitis, NFIP Correspondence,
Human Tests).

48. On Sabin's liability insurance, see Sabin Papers, drawer: Oral Polio Vaccine Production and Human Test, folder: NFIP Insurance, Polio Vaccine Studies.

49. Sabin's consent statement released Sabin himself, the Children's Hospital Research Foundation at the University of Cincinnati, and the U.S. Bureau of Prisons from liability for injury. Initially, the Foundation's legal department told Sabin to leave the organization's name out of the consent document. The legal department then reversed its
position. Stephen Ryan, the general counsel for the Foundation, told Sabin that "it was the
National Foundation's insurer that was desirous of having the Foundation's name in the

consent form." See Albert Sabin to Stephen V. Ryan, January 14, 1955, and Stephen Ryan to Albert Sabin, January 18, 1955, Sabin Papers, drawer: Polio Correspondence and Polio Data, folder: Chillicothe Project–Correspondence.

50. I was unable to locate documents from the animal division of the U.S. Department of Agriculture concerning funds it made available for Stokes's influenza research or from Temple University concerning support that Kolmer received from the institution's Neurology Fund.

51. New York Foundation, *Forty Year Report, 1909–1949* (New York: New York Foundation, n.d.).

52. On the composition of the Rockefeller Institute's scientific board, see Corner, *History of the Rockefeller Institute*, p. 586.

53. Foundation files on IHD projects include numerous evaluations written by Rockefeller Institute scientists.

54. Raymond B. Fosdick, *The Story of the Rockefeller Foundation* (New York: Harper, 1952), p. 293. The statement is italicized in the original. The Foundation also allowed grantees to use funds for activities not originally specified, so long as such use was consistent with the general aims for which the grant was awarded (ibid., pp. 291–92). On the IHD, also see John Farley, *To Cast Out Disease: A History of the International Health Division of Rockefeller Foundation, 1913–1951* (Oxford: Oxford University Press, 2004).

55. Background on Lederle can be found in John R. Wilson, *Margin of Safety* (New York: Doubleday, 1963), and Tom Mahoney, *The Merchants of Life: An Account of the American Pharmaceutical Industry* (New York: Harper, 1959).

56. Wilson, *Margin of Safety*, pp. 142–43.

57. Sociologists have noted that technological mishaps are often associated with faulty information management. Accidents occur when decision makers misperceive risks, when structures or processes impede the communication of information from one unit to another, and when those with authority discount risk assessments made by subordinates or organizational outsiders. See Diane Vaughan, "Regulating Risk: Implications of the Challenger Accident," in *Organizations, Uncertainties, and Risk*, ed. James F. Short and Lee Clarke (Boulder: Westview Press, 1992), pp. 235–53; Diane Vaughan, *The Challenger Launch Decision* (Chicago: University of Chicago Press, 1996); and Barry A. Turner, "The Organizational and Interorganizational Development of Disasters," *Administrative Science Quarterly* 21 (1976): 378–97. For more on information management in organizations, see Arthur L. Stinchcombe, *Information and Organizations* (Berkeley and Los Angeles: University of California Press, 1990).

58. For one overview of the voluminous literature on organizational environments, see Richard W. Scott, *Organizations: Rational, Natural, and Open Systems*, 4th ed. (Englewood Cliffs, N.J.: Prentice-Hall, 1998).

59. Sociological literature includes many descriptions of networks of organizations and interorganizational influence. New institutional theorists offer a number of versions. Paul J. DiMaggio and Walter W. Powell develop the concept of the "organizational field" in "The Iron Cage Revisited: Institutional Isomorphism and Collective Rationality," *American Sociological Review* 48 (1983): 147–60. W. Richard Scott and John W. Meyer develop the notion of "societal sectors" in "The Organization of Societal Sectors: Propositions and Early Evidence," in *New Institutionalism in Organizational Analysis*, ed. Walter W. Powell and Paul

J. DiMaggio (Chicago: University of Chicago Press, 1991), pp. 108–40. The new institutional perspective sees networks of organizations and their normative environments as evolving together. See, for example, Paul J. DiMaggio, "Constructing an Organizational Field as a Professional Project: U.S. Art Museums, 1920–1940," in *New Institutionalism in Organizational Analysis*, ed. Walter W. Powell and Paul J. DiMaggio (Chicago: University of Chicago Press, 1991), pp. 267–92.

60. David L. Sills examines the National Foundation's mobilization of volunteer workers in *The Volunteers: Means and Ends in a National Organization* (Glencoe: Free Press, 1957).

61. Jonathan Liebenau uses the term "scientific entrepreneurialism" in *Medical Science and Medical Industry: The Formation of the American Pharmaceutical Industry* (Baltimore: Johns Hopkins University Press, 1987).

62. On the history of the ICM, see both Liebenau, *Medical Science and Medical Industry*, and "Abstract of Minutes of Meeting of Organization, Dermatological Research Laboratories, Inc.," 1921, by Jay Schamberg, DRL Records, box ZZ8C 46. Available records shed no light on how the ICM's endowment fared during the stock market crash of 1929 and the economic depression of the 1930s.

63. I am grateful to Janet Tighe for information on the ICM's activities during the 1930s. Her forthcoming book on Temple University Medical School is entitled *A "Key of Gold": Medicine, Money, and Public Good in the History of an American Medical School*.

64. I found no evidence that either Kolmer or the ICM were subject to legal suit as a result of polio-vaccine deaths and injuries. Accidents with experimental vaccines fell into a gray area of the law. The ICM distributed Kolmer's vaccine free of charge and labeled it experimental. As discussed in chapter 2, these measures placed the vaccine outside the regulatory scope of the National Institute of Health and may also have given protection to Kolmer and the ICM in the event of product liability action. A medical malpractice suit, if filed, might have been directed toward the physician administering the vaccine. In most cases, this was not Kolmer. Physicians who worked for public health departments were probably protected from suit by the common law tradition of eminent domain, which prohibits damage suits against government agencies. Furthermore, during the 1930s, injured parties would have been discouraged from initiating litigation by the fact that contemporary medical science provided no tools for determining whether a particular case of polio was caused by an unsafe vaccine or by natural exposure to the disease.

65. Kolmer's fate is a striking contrast to that of Park and Brodie, whose vaccine, also used in the mid-1930s, was viewed as safer than Kolmer's. In 1936, Park began a long delayed retirement, and Brodie lost his job at New York University. On the transfer of the ICM's endowment to Temple University, see the four-page typescript "History of the Institute of Public Health and Preventive Medicine of Temple University," by John A. Kolmer, dated July 26, 1954, DRL Records, box 3, folder: Kolmer, John A., 1886–1962.

66. Lederle's expenditures on polio-vaccine development are from Wilson, *Margin of Safety*, p. 136; figure for proceeds from Aureomycin is from Mahoney, *Merchants of Life*, p. 178.

67. On the impact of the Cutter incident—and other contemporary developments— on the companies undertaking vaccine development, see Galambos and Sewell, *Networks of Innovation*, pp. 60–61. The Cutter incident triggered the reorganization of the control of bi-

ologicals within the NIH. See Margaret Pittman, "The Regulation of Biologic Products, 1902–1972," in *National Institute of Allergy and Infectious Disease: Intramural Contributions, 1887–1987*, ed. Harriet R. Greenwald and Victoria A. Harden (Washington, D.C.: National Institutes of Health, 1987). Scientific papers on the Cutter episode include Neal Nathanson and Alexander D. Langmuir, "The Cutter Incident: Poliomyelitis following Formaldehyde-Inactivated Poliovirus Vaccination in the United States during the Spring of 1955," *American Journal of Hygiene* 78 (1963): 16–79. Settlements in Cutter court cases give a sense of the financial consequences, at midcentury, of successfully litigated vaccine injuries. One child, permanently paralyzed after being inoculated with Cutter vaccine, received a settlement of $132,000. Another, less seriously affected, received $16,000. Settlement details are from a clipping from the *San Francisco Chronicle*, Saturday, January 18, 1958, Salk Papers, Polio Files, box 108, folder 7: Cutter Lawsuit.

68. On variability among firms in their willingness to consider product liability suits as a cost of doing business, see Joseph Sanders, "Firm Risk Management in the Face of Product Liability Rules," in Short and Clarke *Organizations, Uncertainty, and Risk*, pp. 57–81.

69. Lee Clarke and James F. Short, "Social Organization and Risk: Some Current Controversies," *Annual Review of Sociology* 19 (1993): 392–93.

70. These measures included announcing that the Rockefeller Institute Hospital would refrain from experiments on patients and instructing authors of articles to be published in the *Journal of Experimental Medicine*, edited by a Rockefeller Institute scientist, to remove language about human experimentation that might trigger antivivisection attacks. On the Rockefeller Institute's early experiences with antivivisection activists, see Susan E. Lederer, "Hideyo Noguchi's Luetin Experiment and the Antivivisectionists," *Isis* 76 (1985): 31–48; Susan E. Lederer, "Political Animals: The Shaping of Biomedical Research Literature in Twentieth-Century America," *Isis* 83 (1992): 61–89; Lederer, *Subjected to Science*.

71. Memo dated April 14, 1954, from the office of Basil O'Connor to "HD [History Department] Staff," NFIP Records, series: Procedures, folder: Vaccine (General).

72. On the importance of organizations to risk management, see Clarke and Short, "Social Organization and Risk"; Lee Clarke, "Explaining Choices among Technological Risks," *Social Problems* 35, no. 1 (1988): 22–35; James Short and Clarke, *Organizations, Uncertainty, and Risk*. Commentary on the field of risk analysis and its rationalization of dangers includes Mary Douglas, *Risk Acceptability according to the Social Sciences* (New York: Russell Sage, 1985). On the social construction of risk and presentations to the public, see Clarke and Short, "Social Organization and Risk"; James F. Short, "The Social Fabric at Risk: Toward the Social Transformation of Risk Analysis," *American Sociological Review* 49 (1984): 711–25; and Lee Clarke, *Mission Improbable: Using Fantasy Documents to Tame Disaster* (Chicago: University of Chicago Press, 1999). Discussions of strategies for containing repercussions of injuries include Craig Calhoun and Henry K. Hiller, "Coping with Insidious Injuries: The Case of Johns-Mansville Corporation and Asbestos Exposure," *Social Problems* 35, no. 2 (April 1988): 162–81; and Elaine Draper, "Preventive Law by Corporate Professional Team Players: Liability and Responsibility in the Work of Company Doctors," *Journal of Contemporary Health Law and Policy* 15 (1999): 525–607.

73. On the paucity of comparative studies of organizational management of risk, see James F. Short Jr. and Lee Clarke, "Social Organization and Risk," in Short and Clarke, *Organizations, Uncertainty, and Risk*, p. 312.

Chapter Four

1. Irvin Stewart describes the CMR's structure in *Organizing Scientific Research for War* (Boston: Little, Brown, 1948), pp. 98–119. On the CMR's relation to the National Research Council, see Rexmond C. Cochrane, *The National Academy of Science: The First Hundred Years, 1863–1963* (Washington D.C.: National Academy of Sciences, 1978), pp. 408–14. For the wide range of research undertaken under CMR sponsorship, see E. Cowles Andrus et al., eds., *Advances in Military Medicine*, 2 vols. (Boston: Little, Brown, 1948).

2. The AEB was constituted in 1941 as the Board for the Investigation and Control of Influenza and Other Epidemic Diseases. It was renamed the Army Epidemiology Board in 1944. See Theodore E. Woodward, *The Armed Forces Epidemiology Board: Its First Fifty Years* (Falls Church, Va.: Office of the Surgeon General, Department of the Army, 1990).

3. Woodward reports funding levels for the AEB (ibid., p. 331). Figures on the CMR funding are found in Andrus et al., *Advances in Military Medicine*, 1:xliii–xliv, and Stewart, *Organizing Scientific Research for War*, pp. 104–5.

4. Chester S. Keefer, "Dr. Richards as Chairman of the Committee on Medical Research," *Annals of Internal Medicine* 71, no. 5 (November 1969), S8:62.

5. David J. Rothman, *Strangers at the Bedside: A History of How Law and Bioethics Transformed Medical Decision Making* (New York: Basic Books, 1991), p. 31.

6. James A. Shannon, "The Advancement of Medical Research: A Twenty-Year View of the Role of the National Institutes of Health," *Journal of Medical Education* 42, no. 2 (February 1967): 97–108.

7. John Rowan Wilson, *Margin of Safety* (New York: Doubleday, 1963), p. 62.

8. Jane S. Smith, "Suspended Judgement: Remembering the Role of Thomas Francis, Jr., in the Design of the 1954 Salk Vaccine Trial," *Controlled Clinical Trials* 13 (1992): 181–84. Other secondary accounts of the Salk field trial include Allan M. Brandt, "Polio, Politics, Publicity, and Duplicity: Ethical Aspects in the Development of the Salk Vaccine," *International Journal of Health Services* 8, no. 2 (1978): 257–70; Allan Chase, *Magic Shots* (New York: William Morrow, 1982), pp. 293–307; Richard Carter, *Breakthrough: The Saga of Jonas Salk* (New York: Trident, 1966); Aaron E. Klein, *Trial by Fury: The Polio Vaccine Controversy* (New York: Scribner's, 1972); Jane S. Smith, *Patenting the Sun: Polio and the Salk Vaccine* (New York: Doubleday, 1990); and Wilson, *Margin of Safety*.

9. Max Weber, *Economy and Society: An Interpretive Sociology*, ed. Guenther Roth and Claus Wittich, vol. 2 (1924; Berkeley and Los Angeles: University of California Press, 1978). On the relationship between organizational size and administrative complexity, see Richard W. Scott, *Organizations: Rational, Natural, and Open Systems*, 4th ed. (Englewood Cliffs, N.J.: Prentice-Hall, 1998), pp. 260–61.

10. Seminal work on new institutionalism includes John W. Meyer and Brian Rowan, "Institutionalized Organizations: Formal Structure as Myth and Ceremony," *American Journal of Sociology* 83 (1977): 340–63; Paul J. DiMaggio and Walter W. Powell, "The Iron Cage Revisited: Institutional Isomorphism and Collective Rationality," *American Sociological Review* 48 (1983): 147–60; John W. Meyer and W. Richard Scott, eds., *Organizational Environments: Ritual and Rationality* (1983; Newbury Park, Calif.: Sage, 1992). Walter W. Powell and Paul J. DiMaggio, eds., *New Institutionalism in Organizational Analysis* (Chicago: University of Chicago Press, 1991).

11. Ruth R. Faden and Tom L. Beauchamp write that "four battery decisions between

1905 and 1914 are almost universally credited with formulating the basic features of consent in American law" (*A History and Theory of Informed Consent* [New York: Oxford University Press, 1986], p. 120). On these cases, also see Allan H. McCoid, "A Reappraisal of Liability for Unauthorized Medical Treatment," *Minnesota Law Review* 41, no. 4 (March 1957):
381–434. The four battery rulings established that a surgeon who operates on a patient
without consent is liable for damages for unauthorized treatment. It was not until the *Salgo*
decision in 1957 (a negligence case) that the court began to specify that consent was to be
informed and began to delineate what that meant.

12. G. Edward White, *Tort Law in America: An Intellectual History* (New York: Oxford
University Press 1980), pp. 147–50. Craig Calhoun and Henry K. Hiller note that, by the
1940s, a shift in the interpretation of tort law allowed use of liability insurance as a means
for redistributing risk and allowing hazardous but socially desirable ventures to be undertaken. See "Coping with Insidious Injuries: The Case of Johns-Manville Corporation and
Asbestos Exposure," *Social Problems* 35, no. 2 (April 1988): 172.

13. Carol A. Heimer notes that in many institutional arenas, insurance has supplanted other forms of risk management. See "Insuring More, Ensuring Less: The Costs
and Benefits of Private Regulation through Insurance," in *Embracing Risk*, ed. Tom Backer
and Jonathan Simon (Chicago: University of Chicago Press, 2002). This has not been the
case with human experimentation.

14. National Commission for the Protection of Human Subjects of Biomedical and Behavioral Research, *The Belmont Report: Ethical Principles and Guidelines for the Protection of
Human Subjects* (Washington, D.C.: U.S. Government Printing Office, 1978).

15. Harvey Cushing, *The Life of Sir William Osler,* vol. 2 (Oxford: Clarendon Press,
1925), p. 109; also cited in Albert R. Jonsen, *The Birth of Bioethics* (New York: Oxford University Press, 1998), p. 131. On the consent statement used in Walter Reed's experiment,
see Advisory Committee on Human Radiation Experiments, *Final Report* (Washington,
D.C.: U.S. Government Printing Office, 1995), p. 97; and Susan E. Lederer, *Subjected to Science: Human Experimentation in America before the Second World War* (Baltimore: Johns
Hopkins University Press, 1995), pp. 21–22.

16. William H. Park to Dr. R. C. Williams, October 22, 1934, PHS Records, General
Files, box 60, folder: Poliomyelitis (emphasis added).

17. Chauncey Starr, "Social Benefit versus Technological Risk," *Science* 165 (September 19, 1969): 1235, 1937.

18. Sydney R. Taber, "Shall Vivisection be Restricted?" letter to the editor, *Chicago
Record-Herald,* May 12, 1905, p. 6; cited in Lederer, *Subjected to Science,* p. 75.

19. Lederer, *Subjected to Science.*

20. Ibid., p. 94; Susan E. Lederer, "Political Animals: The Shaping of Biomedical Research Literature in Twentieth-Century America," *Isis* 83: 1 (1992): 61–79. Also see Saul
Benison, "In Defense of Medical Research," *Harvard Medical Alumni Bulletin* 44, no. 3
(1970): 16–23. Cannon also urged that the AMA amend its ethical codes to require patients' cooperation and consent in the conduct of clinical experiments. Others resisted Cannon's suggestion, fearing that a formal statement about researchers' responsibilities to
subjects would strengthen the antivivisectionists' hand. It was not until December 1946, on
the eve of the Nuremberg trials, that the AMA issued a code of conduct for medical research. This code specified the need for voluntary consent, prior animal studies, and proper

medical protection and management. See *JAMA 132* (December 23, 1946): 1090 and *JAMA* 133 (January 4, 1947): 35; also cited in Advisory Committee on Human Radiation Experiments, *Final Report* (Washington, D.C.: U.S. Government Printing Office, 1995), pp. 135, 165 nn. 15, 16.

21. [Walter Cannon], "The Right and Wrong of Making Experiments on Human Beings," *JAMA* 67, no. 19 (November 4, 1916): 1373.

22. *Schloendorff v. Society of New York Hospitals,* 211 N.Y. 128, 105 N.E. 93 (1914); cited in Faden and Beauchamp, *History and Theory of Informed Consent,* p. 123.

23. Jon H. Harkness, "Research behind Bars: A History of Nontherapeutic Research on American Prisoners" (Ph.D. diss., University of Wisconsin, Madison, 1996), p. 3.

24. Stokes's correspondence with Pennhurst State School in the early 1940s provides insight into contemporary understandings about when consent was considered necessary. In negotiating access to subjects at Pennhurst, Stokes wrote to the institution's director that he had already vaccinated seventy-four children in six institutions plus "other children living privately in Philadelphia . . . which group includes my own child." Stokes continued: "In all cases except Homewood and St. Vincent's, which are the most recent vaccinated groups, we have obtained parental consent, but with the passage of time (having started almost two years ago) we can vouch for the harmlessness and also to a considerable extent for its efficacy. . . . I don't believe at Pennhurst parental consent would be necessary but we would be glad to accede to whatever your judgement on this may be" (Joseph Stokes Jr. to James S. Dean, June 30, 1941, Stokes Papers, box: Measles no. 5, folder: Pennhurst State School).

25. Dean also wrote to Sandy on June 20, 1941: "I can, of course, appreciate the necessity of exercising every possible precaution to avoid anything which might possibly jeopardize the health of the patients or which might subject the Institution to criticism. . . . It occurs to me that if the inoculations have been shown to be of definite value on the basis of a sufficient number of cases, we might be covered from the standpoint of criticism if a letter were addressed to the parents or guardian of each patient, individually, requesting his authorization and explaining the nature of the procedure completely." Both letters are from Stokes Papers, box: Measles no. 5, folder: Pennhurst State School.

26. See, for example, E. L. Johnson, superintendent of Woodbine Colony for Feeble Minded Males, to Stokes's junior collaborator, Gerald O'Neil, September 1, 1939: "We have something over forty children available [for] whom we have parental consent, and who, according to the family history, have not had measles. . . . When the controls are selected, I will have to go, or send someone, to the parents to gain their specific permission for inoculation with the unmodified virus" (Stokes Papers, box: Measles no. 5, folder: Squibb Institute no. 2).

27. A. N. Richards to J. E. Moore, October 9, 1942, OSRD Records, CMR General Records, 1945–46 (series 165), box: 43, folder: Human Experiments–V.D.; also cited in Advisory Committee on Human Radiation Experiments, *Final Report,* p. 97. The context in which Richards made this statement was a discussion of an experiment involving giving gonorrhea to prison inmates. See note 35 below for more on this experiment.

28. For examples of AEB consent documents, see Stokes Papers, box: Measles no. 7, folder: Measles Volunteers no. 1. On the National Foundation's directions to polio researchers regarding consent forms to be used in early human trials, see note 32 below.

Foundation correspondence with Salk and other investigators regarding consent documents can be found in NFIP Records, series: Procedures, folder: Vaccine, Polio, Salk, Consent to Immunize.

29. Consent form accompanying letter of July 31, 1935, from Rockefeller Institute business manager Edric B. Smith to Homer F. Swift at the Rockefeller Institute Hospital, Business Manager's Files, box 14, folder: Influenza, 1918–45.

30. Richard's stipulation is from A. N. Richards to J. E. Moore, October 9, 1942, , OSRD Records, CMR General Records, box: 43, folder: Human Experiments–V.D.; also cited in Advisory Committee on Human Radiation Experiments, *Final Report*, p. 97. Wording of the AEB clause is from "Waiver and Release," dated October 1945, Stokes Papers, box: Measles no. 7, folder: Measles Volunteers no. 1.

31. Drafts of consent statements to be used in early trials of Salk's polio strains include no waiver clauses. See NFIP Records, series: Procedures, folder: Vaccine, Polio, Salk, Consent to Immunize. The consent document used later in the large-scale field trial of Salk's vaccine also had no waiver provision. See Thomas Francis Jr., "Appendix E," in *Evaluation of the 1954 Field Trial of Poliomyelitis Vaccine: Final Report* (Ann Arbor: Poliomyelitis Vaccine Evaluation Center, Department of Epidemiology, School of Public Health, University of Michigan, 1957), p. 460.

32. One in-house critic observed that a draft consent document for the Salk vaccine field trial was "singularly lacking in appreciation of public attitudes toward such studies. While legally it may be satisfying, I am sure that were I, as a parent, to be the recipient of such a document, I would tell both the Foundation and the investigator exactly were they could go. I think it is exceedingly cold, lacking in appreciation of what a parent feels when called upon to make such a decision." The commentator advised that the wording of consent forms should avoid legalisms and be "simple, direct and clear." See National Foundation internal memo dated December 4, 1953, from Morton Seidenfeld, director of public education, to Melvin Glasser, assistant to the Foundation's president. Earlier, in the course of developing a consent statement for use in testing his vaccine at Polk State School, Jonas Salk wrote to Harry M. Weaver, the Foundation's director of research, regarding feedback from the school's physician-director: "Although he agreed that the legal and scientific requirements were met by the form as submitted, it is his feeling that it does not meet the psychological requirements for facilitating his part of the job"—which was getting parents to sign the form. Salk recommended revising the consent statement "to make it seem less legal." See Jonas E. Salk to Harry M. Weaver, May 17, 1952. Both the internal memo and the letter can be found in the NFIP Records, series: Procedures, folder: Vaccine, Polio, Salk, Consent to Immunize. This folder contains records documenting extensive communications about the consent statements used in Salk's early trials.

33. Albert Sabin to Stephen V. Ryan, January 14, 1955, and Stephen Ryan to Albert Sabin, January 18, 1955; both letters in Sabin Papers, drawer: Polio Correspondence and Polio Data; folder: Chillicothe Project–Correspondence.

34. These documents also included waiver clauses. The wording regarding provision of medical care is as follows: "It is expressly understood and agreed that notwithstanding this Waiver and Release, said Board and Commission will furnish medical and hospital care for any acute illness which I may have as a direct result of the aforesaid experiment, it being understood that said Commission or its members or agents shall be the sole judge as to whether or not any illness is sufficiently acute to require such medical or hospital care

and of the duration thereof" ("Waiver and Release," dated November 1945, Stokes Papers, box: Measles no. 7, folder: Measles Volunteers no. 1).

35. A. N. Richards to J. E. Moore, October 31, 1942, , OSRD Records, CMR General Correspondence, Human Experiments–Venereal Disease, box 39; also cited in Rothman, *Strangers at the Bedside*, p. 44. The gonorrhea-prophylaxis experiment was begun but never completed because researchers were unable to develop a reliable method for producing the clinical disease in volunteers. For discussion of the experiment and surrounding debate at the CMR, see Harkness, "Research behind Bars," pp. 87–101; Harry M. Marks, "Where Do Ethics Come From? The Case of Human Experimentation" (paper delivered at the Center for Biomedical Ethics, Case Western Reserve University, March 1988); Harry M. Marks, *The Progress of Experiment* (New York: Cambridge University Press, 1997), pp. 101–5; Rothman, *Strangers at the Bedside*, pp. 42–47.

36. Harkness, "Research behind Bars," pp. 79–87.

37. Robert J. O'Connor, chief of the Legal Office of the Army Surgeon General, to Col. Frank L. Bauer, Army Medical Research and Development Board, October 23, 1947, AFEB Records, entry 14, file: Commission on Liver Disease–Human Volunteers for Hepatitis Studies–Feb. 1948 on; document reprinted in Advisory Committee on Human Radiation Experiments, *Final Report*, supplemental vol. 1 (Washington, D.C.: U.S. Government Printing Office, 1995), p. 92.

38. Letters from Henry W. Kumm, National Foundation director of research, to Albert Sabin on March 22, 1954, and April 20, 1954, Sabin Papers, drawer: Oral Polio Vaccine Production and Human Testing, folder: Poliomyelitis, NFIP Correspondence, Human Tests. Kumm was referring to initial human tests of Salk's killed-virus vaccine, not to the large-scale field trial of the vaccine that was about to begin. Howard A. Howe, a researcher at Johns Hopkins, describes his trial of polio strains in National Foundation for Infantile Paralysis, *Proceedings of the Committee on Immunization*, December 4, 1951, pp. 36–43, NFIP Materials, Cincinnati Medical Heritage Center.

39. Memo dated April 22, 1954, from Basil O'Connor, National Foundation president, to "All Grantees of the NFIP": "In the development of any preventive or therapeutic measure to combat poliomyelitis there comes a time when preliminary trials, previously carried out in experimental animals, must [be] extended to human beings. To individuals of the caliber of grantees supported by the National Foundation for Infantile Paralysis it hardly seems necessary to urge unusual precaution and careful thought before taking such a momentous step. My duty, however, compels me, in addition, to advise you that the National Foundation would be subject to suit in the event of any unfortunate accidents occurring as a result of human vaccinations. Precedents already established by this organization in the cases of Dr. Howard Howe and Dr. Jonas Salk involved adequate arrangements for accident as well as for health insurance coverage. For those reasons we are requesting that you advise the National Foundation well in advance, whenever you plan to carry out human trials, particularly with a potential vaccine or a new immunizing agent" (Sabin Papers, drawer: Oral Polio Vaccine Production and Human Testing, folder: Poliomyelitis, NFIP Correspondence, Human Tests).

40. Albert Sabin to Stephen Ryan of the National Foundation's legal department, January 14, 1955, Rivers Papers, folder: Sabin, Albert, no. 1. Records of Sabin's insurance policies are found in the Sabin Papers, drawer: Oral Polio Vaccine Production and Human Tests, folder: Polio NFIP, Insurance, Polio Vaccine Studies.

41. Cecil J. Watson, director of the AEB Commission on Liver Disease and a faculty member at the University of Minnesota, asked two colleagues, one the dean of his university's law school and the other an expert in criminology, whether a waiver form would indeed protect against liability claims. In a letter dated April 5, 1948, Watson reported the results of his inquiry to Dr. Colin M. MacLeod, AEB president and a faculty member at New York University School of Medicine: "I asked them specifically whether a waiver signed by volunteers would be legal at a later date, insofar as avoidance of responsibility for disability or death was concerned. I asked this question with respect to a waiver made out to the individual experimenter as well as to one assigned to the official agency sponsoring the research, that is to say, the Army Epidemiology Board of the War Department. They did not believe that such a waiver would be of much value, although they stated that so far as they knew there was no precedent in law to determine in advance what might happen in case of a suit. They pointed out that a clever attorney at some later date might very well be able to overthrow such a waiver and get a judgment against an experimenter in case of a disability or even succeed in having him declared guilty of homicide in case of death. . . . According to my legal friends . . . responsibility for . . . experiments [currently being considered] would devolve entirely upon the individual experimenter in case of a later suit or complaint" (AFEB Records, entry 14, folder: Commission on Liver Disease–Human Volunteers for Hepatitis Studies–Feb. 1948 on; document reprinted in Advisory Committee on Human Radiation Experiments, *Final Report*, supplemental vol. 1, pp. 136–37).

42. Irving Ladimer, "Law and Medicine, a Symposium: Ethical and Legal Aspects of Medical Research on Human Beings," *Journal of Public Law* 3, no. 1 (spring 1954): 509. Ladimer also doubted that waiver provisions would hold up in court. While his published remarks do not indicate whom he is referring to by "responsible organizations," archival records indicate that Ladimer interviewed National Foundation research staff about their oversight practices in the spring of 1953. See NFIP Records, series: Government Relations (Federal), folder: NIH 1944.

43. It may be that liability insurance for medical researchers was being handled as a feature of their employment. During the early 1960s, the Boston University Law-Medicine Research Institute surveyed eighty-six departments of medicine, receiving fifty-two responses. When asked about liability insurance, twenty-three departments indicated that either the institution or its researchers were covered by liability insurance. See "Summary Report of Two Questionnaire Surveys," *Final Report of Administrative Practices in Clinical Research* (Boston: Law-Medicine Research Institute, Boston University, 1963), p. 14; William C. Curran, "Government Regulation of the Use of Human Subjects in Medical Research: The Approach of Two Federal Agencies," in *Experimentation with Human Subjects*, ed. Paul A. Freund (New York: George Braziller, 1970), p. 407.

44. For a statement of this NIH policy, see the memorandum dated December 17, 1953, to "Those Concerned" from John Trautman, director of the NIH Clinical Center, entitled "Group Consideration of Clinical Research Procedures Deviating from Accepted Medical Practice or Involving Unusual Hazards" (NIH-OD Files, subject category: Research, folder: Research 3–Clinical Investigation, 1953–80, document no. 010191). On disagreements within NIH's Clinical Research Committee about the boundaries between experimental and "accepted" practice, see Harry Marks, "Where Do Ethics Come From? The Role of Disciplines and Institutions" (paper delivered at the Conference on Ethical Issues in Clinical Trials, University of Alabama at Birmingham, February 25–26, 2000).

45. Memorandum, dated May 11, 1953, entitled "Principles and Practices of the National Foundation for Infantile Paralysis: Human Research," from Irving Ladimer to Dr. Russell M. Wilder, NFIP Records, series: Government Relations (Federal), folder: NIH 1944. At that time, Wilder chaired an informal committee at NIH on human experimentation in clinical settings. Mention of Wilder's committee is from Irving Ladimer to Harry Weaver, April 22, 1953, NFIP Records, series: Government Relations (Federal), folder: NIH 1944.

46. In 1953, the National Foundation's Immunization Committee was split over the preferability of a killed or live vaccine. Jane Smith writes that Basil O'Connor circumvented that committee when arranging for approval of the Salk field trials. O'Connor, she writes, "was convinced there would never be certainty sufficient for the cautious, disputatious experts" on the Immunization Committee. O'Connor solved the problem by setting up the smaller Vaccine Advisory Committee. See Smith, *Patenting the Sun*, pp. 192–93. For another account of the creation of the Vaccine Advisory Committee, see Saul Benison, *Tom Rivers: Reflections on a Life of Medicine and Science* (Cambridge: MIT Press, 1967), pp. 502–4.

47. On the review of Sabin's protocol, see chapter 3 above.

48. Of the fifty-two departments of medicine responding to the survey from the Boston University Law-Medicine Research Institute, twenty-two indicated that they provided peer review of research protocols on an advisory basis. See "Summary Report of Two Questionnaire Surveys," pp. 8–9; also cited in Rothman, *Strangers at the Bedside*, p. 60. On the University of Washington's board, see Diane J. McCann and John R. Pettit, "A Report on Adverse Effects of Insurance for Human Subjects," in *Compensating for Research Injuries*, vol. 2, *Appendices*, ed. President's Commission for the Study of Ethical Problems in Medical and Biomedical and Behavioral Research (Washington D.C.: U.S. Government Printing Office, 1982), p. 241. Harry Marks discusses the committee at Johns Hopkins in "Where Do Ethics Come From? The Role of Disciplines and Institutions." Marks notes that the Hopkins committee focused on methodological issues rather than ethical ones.

49. DiMaggio and Powell use the term "normative isomorphism" to refer to the importation of practices from societal rule carriers and the term "mimetic isomorphism" to refer to imitation of the practices of other organizations. See "The Iron Cage Revisited."

50. On organizational responses to ambiguous legal mandates, see Lauren B. Edelman, "Legal Environments and Organizational Governance: The Expansion of Due Process in the American Workplace," *American Journal of Sociology* 95 (1990): 1401–40; Lauren B. Edelman, "Legal Ambiguity and Symbolic Structures: Organizational Mediation of Law," *American Journal of Sociology* 97 (1992): 1530–76; Frank R. Dobbin, Lauren B. Edelman, John W. Meyer, and W. Richard Scott, "Equal Opportunity Law and the Construction of Internal Labor Markets," *American Journal of Sociology* 99 (1993): 396–427; Mark C. Suchman and Lauren B. Edelman, "Legal Rational Myth: The New Institutionalism and the Law and Society Tradition," *Law and Social Inquiry* 21, no. 4 (fall 1996): 903–41; Lauren B. Edelman and Mark C. Suchman, "The Legal Environment of Organizations," *Annual Review of Sociology* 23 (1997): 479–515. For further elaboration of the importance of professionals in constructing and disseminating strategies for legal compliance, see Lauren B. Edelman, Steven E. Abraham, and Howard S. Erlanger, "Professional Construction of Law: The Inflated Threat of Wrongful Discharge," *Law and Society Review* 25, no. 1 (1992): 47–83; John R. Sutton and Frank Dobbin, "The Two Faces of Governance: Responses to Legal Un-

certainty in U.S. Firms, 1955 to 1985," *American Sociological Review* 61 (1996): 794–811; Bruce G. Carruthers and Terence C. Halliday, *Rescuing Business: The Making of Corporate Bankruptcy Law in England and the United States* (Oxford: Clarendon Press, 1998); and Lauren B. Edelman, Christopher Uggen, and Howard S. Erlanger, "The Endogeneity of Legal Regulation: Grievance Procedures as Rational Myth," *American Journal of Sociology* 105 (1999): 406–54. Carol A. Heimer argues that the professions most central to organizational routines have the greatest impact in shaping whether and how organizations import legal mandates. See "Explaining Variation in the Impact of Law: Organizations, Institutions, and Professions," *Studies in Law, Politics, and Society* 15 (1996): 29–59.

51. Curran, "Government Regulation of the Use of Human Subjects." On the handful of eighteenth-, nineteenth-, and early-twentieth-century malpractice cases in the United States and Britain involving alleged experiments—that is, departures from conventional medical practice—see Elwyn L. Cady Jr., "Medical Malpractice: What about Experimentation?" *Annals of Western Medicine and Surgery* 6 (1952): 164–70; Ladimer, "Law and Medicine"; and Curran, "Government Regulation of the Use of Human Subjects."

52. *Fortner v. Koch* 272 Mich. 273, 261 N.W. 762 (1935); quotation from 261 N.W., p. 265. For commentary on this case, see Curran, "Government Regulation of the Use of Human Subjects," pp. 402–5; and Faden and Beauchamp, *History and Theory of Informed Consent*, p. 191 n. 8.

53. Rockefeller Institute managers discussed the potential for liability associated with Francis's 1935 influenza experiment. See Business Manager's Files, series 210.3, box 14, folder: Influenza, 1918–45. The National Foundation addressed liability issues in letters and memos to polio-vaccine researchers. See, for example, note 39 above. Harkness recounts discussion of potential for liability raised by the OSRD's gonorrhea-prophylaxis experiment in Harkness, "Research behind Bars," p. 94. On relevant communications among AEB commissioners, see note 41 above.

54. Ladimer, "Law and Medicine," p. 473. Ladimer continued: "Legal representatives were active following the death of a laboratory technician at the University of South Dakota from an overdose of an experimental drug and following the death of a federal prisoner at Lewisburg, Pennsylvania, from an injection of hepatitis virus."

55. Curran, "Government Regulation of the Use of Human Subjects," pp. 402–3. By "reported court actions," Curran was apparently referring to appellate decisions. He would likely not have located nonappellate cases or cases settled out of court. As noted in chapter 3, the 1955 Cutter incident—in which 260 contracted polio from insufficiently inactivated batches of the Salk vaccine—involved an approved immunizing agent and thus was not a research accident.

56. On preventive measures taken by other types of organizations when faced with the possibility of legal liability, see Craig Calhoun and Henry K. Hiller, "Coping with Insidious Injuries," pp. 162–81; and Elaine Draper, "Preventive Law by Corporate Professional Team Players: Liability and Responsibility in the Work of Company Doctors," *Journal of Contemporary Health Law and Policy* 15 (1999): 525–607. These authors report that one organizational response to the threat of suit is to withhold information that might be of use to plaintiffs.

57. The Columbia-Presbyterian consent form accompanies a letter from A. E. Dochez to Homer F. Swift, June 14, 1935, Business Manager's Files, box 14, folder: Influenza,

1918–45. Salk forwarded Stokes a consent document "of the type . . . sent to [Salk] by Dr. Weaver" with a letter dated November 6, 1952, Stokes Papers, folder: Salk, Jonas, no. 4. In a letter dated November 14, 1952, Stokes sent Salk (and copied Weaver) a consent form developed at the Philadelphia Serum Exchange by a lawyer on the Board of Managers (NFIP Records, series: Procedures, folder: Vaccine, Polio, Salk, Consent to Immunize). All of these documents included waiver provisions.

58. Albert Sabin to Stephen Ryan, January 14, 1955, Sabin Papers, drawer: Polio Correspondence and Polio Data, folder: Chillicothe Project–Correspondence. The NIII form, like Sabin's, included a waiver provision. See Sabin Papers, drawer: Oral Polio Vaccine Procedures, Human Test, folder: Poliomyelitis NFIP, Chillicothe Blank Release Forms.

59. On nontherapeutic human experiments conducted under federal auspices during and after World War II, see Advisory Committee on Human Radiation Experiments, *Final Report*, and Jonathan D. Moreno, *Undue Risk: Secret State Experiments on Humans* (New York: W. H. Freeman, 1999). Although medical experiments sponsored by the OSRD and the AEB were not secret, many of those sponsored by the Atomic Energy Commission were.

60. Meyer and Rowan, "Institutionalized Organizations."

61. [Cannon,] "The Right and Wrong of Making Experiments on Human Beings," p. 1373.

62. Rothman, *Strangers at the Bedside*.

63. Benison, "In Defense of Medical Research," p. 19 and n. 19.

64. On William Randolph Hearst's antivivisection sympathies and his papers' editorial policies, see Lederer, "Political Animals," p. 63.

65. In 1942, Rous asked Thomas Francis Jr., who had worked at the Rockefeller Institute through 1935, to withdraw a manuscript. The paper causing Rous problems discussed AEB-funded research in which Francis exposed mental patients—some previously immunized and some not—to unmodified influenza virus to test the effectiveness of a vaccine. As Rous put it to Francis: "It may save much trouble if you will publish your paper . . . elsewhere than in the *Journal of Experimental Medicine*. The *Journal* is under constant scrutiny by the antivivisectionists, who would not hesitate to play up the fact that you used for your tests human beings of a state institution. That these tests were wholly justified goes without saying" (Peyton Rous to Thomas Francis Jr., November 16, 1942, Rous Papers, folder: *Journal of Experimental Medicine*–Francis, Thomas).

66. Lederer, "Political Animals," p. 76. Whatever the reality of subjects' participation, "volunteer" invoked the picture of a knowledgeable and consenting subject, willingly choosing to contribute to medical science. In "Research behind Bars," Jon Harkness comments that early-twentieth-century prison researchers routinely used the term "volunteer" when referring to subjects, even in professional correspondence.

67. Sydney A. Halpern, "Constructing Moral Boundaries: Public Discourse on Human Experimentation in Twentieth-Century America," in *Bioethics in Social Context*, ed. Barry C. Hoffmaster (Philadelphia: Temple University Press, 2000), pp. 69–89.

68. G. D. Fairbairn to Stanhope Bayne-Jones, February 14, 1945, and Stanhope Bayne-Jones to G. D. Fairbairn, February 16, 1945, OSG Records, entry 31, zone I, decimal 334 (Boards 1941–46), box 676, folder: Commission on Viral and Rickettsial Diseases: Jaundice Publications.

69. "Next to conducting well its technical work, nothing is more important to the Na-

tional Foundation than its public relations" (Memo from Basil O'Connor to "All Department Heads," July 16, 1945, cited in "Public Relations, 1945–1949," Monograph no. 26, prepared for the Historical Division of the National Foundation for Infantile Paralysis, by Howard Kaminsky, August 1956, p. 43, NFIP Materials, Cincinnati Medical Heritage Center). "It cannot be doubted that O'Connor, Morgan, and behind them Roosevelt were acutely aware of the importance of good press in getting the Foundation started. Important official steps taken by the Foundation, like the establishment of the organization's medical advisory committees . . . were always carefully planned to get maximum public impact" (cited in "Administrative Problems and Changes, 1944–53," Monograph no. 55, prepared for the Historical Division of the National Foundation for Infantile Paralysis by John Storck, December 1956, p. 96, NFIP Materials, Cincinnati Medical Heritage Center).

70. In 1946, the Professional Relations Bureau was established within the Foundation's medical department; in 1947, scientific public relations was moved to this new department. See Kaminsky, "Public Relations, 1945–1949," pp. 13–20. On the growth of the National Foundation's public relations department, see Storck, "Administrative Problems and Changes, 1944–53," p. 100.

71. Francis, "Appendix E," in *Evaluation of the 1954 Field Trial of Poliomyelitis Vaccine*, p. 460. Also see Smith, *Patenting the Sun*, p. 237, and Wilson, *Margin of Safety*, p. 86.

72. Marie S. Winokur, superintendent of Homewood School, to Joseph Stokes Jr., November 7, 1940, Stokes Papers, box: Measles no. 5, folder: Squibb Institute no. 7.

73. Statement for the files from J. B. Donovan, subject: Human Experimentation in Gonorrhea, OSRD Records, CMR General Records, 1940–46 (series 165), box 43, folder: Human Experiments–V.D.; also cited in Harkness, "Research behind Bars," p. 94.

74. On activities of the NSMR, see *Bulletin of the National Society for Medical Research* and Thurman S. Grafton, "The Founding and Early History of the National Society for Medical Research," *Laboratory Animal Science* 30, no. 4 (August 1980): 759–64. Dorothy Nelkin discusses public relations efforts by postwar scientific associations in *Selling Science* (New York: W. H. Freeman, 1995). Kelly Moore suggests that public-interest organizations sometimes mediate the scientific community's relations with the public. See "Organizing Integrity: American Science and the Creation of Public Interest Organizations, 1955–1975," *American Journal of Sociology* 101, no. 6 (May 1996): 1592–1627. On public images of American science, see Marcel C. LaFollette, *Making Science Our Own: Public Images of Science, 1910–1955* (Chicago: University of Chicago Press, 1990); Chrisopher P. Toumey, *Conjuring Science: Scientific Symbols and Cultural Meanings in American Life* (New Brunswick: Rutgers University Press, 1996).

75. Mary Douglas discusses the emergence of the field of risk analysis in *Risk Acceptability according to the Social Sciences* (New York: Russell Sage, 1985). On organizational reliance on risk professionals, see Thomas. M. Dietz and Robert W. Rycroft, *The Risk Professionals* (New York: Sage, 1987). Dietz and Rycroft note (p. 101) that risk professions interact frequently with potential political advisories. Lee Clarke discusses ritual planning in *Mission Improbable: Using Fantasy Documents to Tame Disaster* (Chicago: University of Chicago Press, 1999).

76. On the malleability of risk assessments and the social construction of risk acceptability, see Mary Douglas and Aaron Wildavsky, *Risk and Culture* (Berkeley and Los Angeles: University of California Press, 1982); Lee Clarke and James F. Short Jr., "Social Organi-

zation and Risk: Some Current Controversies," *Annual Review of Sociology* 19 (1993): 375–99. William R. Freudenburg addresses issues of trust in "Risk and Recreancy: Weber, the Division of Labor, and the Rationality of Risk Perception," *Social Forces* 71, no. 4 (June 1993): 909–32. Other treatments of the construction and management of risk in modern society include Ulrich Beck, *Risk Society: Toward a New Modernity* (London: Sage, 1992); Sheila Jasanoff, *Risk Management and Political Culture* (New York: Russell Sage, 1986); Deborah Lupton, *Risk* (London: Routledge, 2003); and Niklas Luhmann, *Risk: A Sociological Theory* (New York: Aldine de Gruyter, 1993).

77. James F. Short Jr. remarks that "the influence of the mass media in public perceptions of risks has been much discussed but little researched" ("The Social Fabric at Risk: Toward the Social Transformation of Risk Analysis," *American Sociological Review* 49 [1984]: 720). For one account of processes underlying the construction of problems within public arenas, see Stephen Hilgartner and Charles L. Bosk, "The Rise and Fall of Social Problems: A Public Arenas Model," *American Journal of Sociology* 94, no. 1 (July 1988): 53–78.

Chapter Five

1. Henry K. Beecher, "Ethics and Clinical Research," *New England Journal of Medicine* 74 (1966): 1354–60.

2. David J. Rothman discusses this World War II ethos in *Strangers at the Bedside: A History of How Law and Bioethics Transformed Medical Decision Making* (New York: Basic Books, 1991).

3. On the generalization of rights, see Paul Starr, *The Social Transformation of American Medicine* (New York: Basic Books, 1982), and Sydney Halpern, "Medical Authority and the Culture of Rights," *Journal of Health Politics, Policy and Law* 29, nos. 4–5 (2004). Deborah Stone points to a shift in emphasis from collective good to individual rights in several arenas of public health policy. See "The Resistible Rise of Preventive Medicine," in *Health Policy in Transition*, ed. Lawrence D. Brown (Durham: Duke University Press, 1987), pp. 103–28.

4. Ruth R. Faden and Tom L. Beauchamp, *A History and Theory of Informed Consent* (New York: Oxford University Press, 1986), pp. 125–32.

5. For a brief description of these experiments, see ibid., pp. 161–67.

6. On rules for consent during the early twentieth century, see the introduction above and Susan E. Lederer, *Subjected to Science: Human Experimentation in America before the Second World War* (Baltimore: Johns Hopkins University Press, 1995).

7. The distinction between both experiment and therapy and experiment and observation would remain problematic.

8. On precedents for rules governing consent incorporated in federal regulatory code, see Robert J. Levine, *Ethics and Regulation of Clinical Research* (Baltimore: Urban and Schwarzenberg, 1986).

9. Mark S. Frankel addresses the role of NIH leadership in shaping federal regulation of experiments with human subjects in "The Development of Policy Guidelines Governing Human Experimentation in the United States: A Case Study of Public Policy-Making for Science and Technology," *Ethics in Science and Medicine* 2 (1975): 43–59; and "Public Policy Making for Biomedical Research: The Case of Human Experimentation" (Ph.D. diss., George Washington University, 1976).

10. Emile Durkheim, *Division of Labor in Society* (1893; New York: Free Press, 1964).

11. William Goode, "Community within a Community: The Professions," *American Sociological Review* 22 (1957): 194–200; Warren O. Hagstrom, *The Scientific Community* (New York: Basic Books, 1965); Charles L. Bosk, *Forgive and Remember: Managing Medical Failure* (Chicago: University of Chicago Press, 1979). For analytic review of work on social control of medical practice, see Charles L. Bosk, "Social Control and Physicians: The Oscillation of Cynicism and Idealism in Sociological Theory," in *Social Controls in the Medical Profession*, ed. Judith Swazey and Stephen Scher (Boston: Oelgeschlager, Gunn & Hain, 1985), pp. 31–51; Dorothy Nelkin, "Social Controls in the Changing Context of Science," in Swazey and Scher, *Social Controls in the Medical Profession*, pp. 83–94; Harriet Zuckerman, "Deviant Behavior and Social Control in Science," in *Deviance and Social Change*, ed. Edward Sagarin (Beverly Hills: Sage, 1977), pp. 87–138.

12. Eliot Freidson, *Profession of Medicine* (New York: Harper and Row, 1970); Eliot Freidson, *Doctoring Together* (New York: Elsevier, 1975).

13. Thomas F. Gieryn, "Boundary-Work and the Demarcation of Science from Non-Science: Strains and Interests in Professional Ideologies of Scientists," *American Sociological Review* 48 (December 1983): 781–95; Thomas F. Gieryn, *Cultural Boundaries of Science: Credibility on the Line* (Chicago: University of Chicago Press, 1999). Michèle Lamont and Virag Molnar discuss more general uses of the concept of boundaries in "The Study of Boundaries in the Social Sciences," *Annual Review of Sociology* 28 (August 2002): 157–95.

14. For a general discussion of organizations' efforts to affect the environment, see Richard W. Scott, *Organizations: Rational, Natural, and Open Systems*, 4th ed. (Englewood Cliffs, N.J.: Prentice-Hall, 1998). On organizational networks that shape national policy agendas, see Edward O. Laumann and David Knoke, *The Organizational State: Social Choice in National Policy Domains* (Madison: University of Wisconsin Press, 1987). On the effect of the law on organizational policy and visa versa, see Bruce C. Carruthers and Terrance C. Halliday, *Rescuing Business: The Making of Corporate Bankruptcy Law in England and the United States* (Oxford: Clarendon Press, 1998); and Lauren B. Edelman, Christopher Uggen, and Howard S. Erlanger, "The Endogeneity of Legal Regulation: Grievance Procedures as Rational Myth," *American Journal of Sociology* 105 (1999): 406–54.

15. Bert Hansen, "America's First Medical Breakthrough: How Popular Excitement about French Rabies Cure in 1885 Raised New Expectations for Medical Progress," *American Historical Review* 103 (April 1998): 373–418; Bert Hansen, "New Images of a New Medicine: Visual Evidence for the Widespread Popularity of Therapeutic Discoveries in America after 1885," *Bulletin of the History of Medicine* 73, no. 4 (winter 1999): 629–78.

16. For citations to social science literatures on risk, see chapter 3, notes 72 and 73, and chapter 4, notes 75 and 76.

17. Institutional theorists have used the term "regulatory regimes" to refer to systems of organizational and legal controls that, they argue, arise within societal sectors. Mark Suchman and Lauren Edelman comment that "studies of regulatory regimes are only in their infancy." Among the issues to be further explored, they continue, is how coherent normative and cognitive structures develop. See "Legal Rational Myths: The New Institutionalism and the Law and Society Tradition," *Law and Social Inquiry* 21, no. 4 (fall 1996): 927–28. The present volume can be understood as an analysis of the early history of a regulatory regime.

18. Ross E. Cheit, *Setting Safety Standards: Regulation in the Public and Private Sectors* (Berkeley and Los Angeles: University of California Press, 1990); Clarke C. Havighurst, "The Place of Private Accreditation among the Instruments of Government," *Law and Contemporary Problems* 57, no. 4 (1995): 1–14; Joseph J. Hinchliffe, "Anticipatory Democracy: The Influence of the Imagined Public on Safety Regulation" (Ph.D. diss., University of Illinois at Urbana-Champaign, 2002); Colin Scott, "Private Regulation of the Public Sector: A Neglected Facet of Contemporary Governance," *Journal of Law and Society* 29, no. 1 (2002): 56–76. Some scholars use the term "communitarian regulation" to depict oversight systems—like that in the nuclear-power industry—where the regulator is closely integrated with the regulated. Joseph V. Rees argues that this type of regulation has three elements: a well-defined industrial morality, communal pressures backing the morality, and institutionalized responsibilities among members. See Rees's *Hostages of Each Other: The Transformation of Nuclear Safety since Three Mile Island* (Chicago: University of Chicago Press, 1994).

19. Lawrence K. Altman, *Who Goes First? The Story of Self-Experimentation in Medicine* (New York: Random House, 1986).

20. "Self-experimentation and use of Public Health Service personnel as subjects in clinical investigation are prohibited, unless prior written consent is granted by the Director of the National Institutes of Health" (from the memorandum dated December 17, 1953, to "Those Concerned" from John Trautman, director of the NIH Clinical Center, entitled, "Group Consideration of Clinical Research Procedures Deviating from Accepted Medical Practice or Involving Unusual Hazards," NIH-OD Files, subject category: research, folder: Research 3—Clinical Investigation, 1953–80, document no. 010191).

21. In 1932, Flexner and Peyton Rous intervened when a scientist made a public statement critical of Pasteur's investigatory conduct that they viewed as potential ammunition for regulatory activists. On this incident, see my discussion in chapter 3.

22. One rancorous dispute concerned the series of experiments conducted by Saul Krugman at Willowbrook. Beginning in 1956, Krugman infected hundreds of institutionalized children with hepatitis in an effort to prove the existence of two distinct strains of the virus and to develop a hepatitis vaccine. In the spring and summer of 1971, the leading British medical journal, *Lancet*, published commentary on Krugman's studies including numerous letters condemning his conduct. Intraprofessional conflict centered on whether parental consent for Krugman's experiments was voluntary, and whether, even with voluntary parental consent, it is ethically acceptable to use children as subjects in experiments unrelated to their own medical treatment. Editorial policy at both *JAMA* and the *New England Journal of Medicine* supported Krugman's methods.

23. Renée C. Fox and Judith P. Swazey, *Spare Parts: Organ Replacement in American Society* (New York: Oxford University Press, 1992), pp. 23–24.

24. On the impact of law on bioethics, see Rothman, *Strangers at the Bedside*. On the consequences of social movements for investigatory policies, see Steven Epstein, *Impure Science: AIDS, Activism, and the Politics of Knowledge* (Berkeley and Los Angeles: University of California Press, 1996). For one view of the fate of bioethical debate in public arenas, see John H. Evans, *Playing God: Human Genetic Engineering and the Rationalization of Public Bioethical Debate* (Chicago: University of Chicago Press, 2002).

25. Stephen Hilgartner and Charles L. Bosk, "The Rise and Fall of Social Problems: A Public Arenas Model," *American Journal of Sociology* 94, no. 1 (July 1988): 53–78.

Chapter Six

1. Figure on the IHGT's budget from Sheryl Gay Stolbert, "The Biotech Death of Jesse Gelsinger," *New York Times*, November 29, 1999.

2. Kathryn Zoon, head of the CBER, discusses the numbers of gene-therapy protocols and adenovirus-vector protocols in National Institutes of Health, Office of Recombinant DNA Activities (now the Office of Biotechnology Activities), Recombinant DNA Advisory Committee, Minutes of Symposium and Meeting, December 8–10, 1999, p. 23. The minutes of this and other RAC meetings are posted on the RAC Web site at http://www4.od .nih.gov/oba/rac/meetings.html. Hereafter I refer to these documents as "RAC Minutes," identified by the meeting date.

3. The FDA detailed regulatory findings in warning letters issued in 2000 to Batshaw, Raper, and Wilson. These letters are posted on the FDA Web site at http://www.fda.gov/ cber/reading.htm. See, for example, the twenty-page letter to Wilson dated March 3, 2000, from Steven Masiello, the director of the Office of Compliance and Biologics Quality within the FDA's Center for Biologics Evaluation and Research (CBER). Newspaper accounts of the FDA's preliminary findings include Rick Weiss and Deborah Nelson, "Method Faulted in Fatal Gene Therapy," *Washington Post*, December 9, 1999; and Sheryl Gay Stolbert, "FDA Officials Fault Penn Team in Gene Therapy Death," *New York Times*, December 9, 1999. Press coverage of FDA warning letters include Rick Weiss and Deborah Nelson, "FDA Lists Violations by Gene Therapy Director at U-Penn," *Washington Post*, March 4, 2000.

4. Quotation from the letter dated July 19, 2001, from Patrick McNeilly and Michael Carome of the U.S. Office of Human Research Protections to administrators at Johns Hopkins School of Medicine, including Edward D. Miller, dean and chief executive officer; Chi Van Dang, vice dean for research; and Gregory Schaffer, president of the Johns Hopkins Bayview Medical Center. This and other OHRP determination letters available on the OHRP Web site at http://ohrp.osophs.dhhs.gov/detrm/index.htm.

5. Robert Steinbrook, "Protecting Research Subjects: The Crisis at Johns Hopkins," *New England Journal of Medicine* 346, no. 9 (2002): 719. Nearly two years after Roche's death, the FDA's Center for Drug Evaluation and Research (CDER) took action against Togias with a warning letter issued on March 31, 2003. This letter can be found on the CDER's Web site at http://www.fda.gov/cder/warn/. A spokesman for Johns Hopkins University stated that the CDER proposed placing unspecified restricts on Togias's investigatory activities. The spokesman indicated also that Togias's research project had restarted and that CDER restrictions would be "limited" (Julie Bell, "JHU Researcher Found To Have Violated Rules, FDA Proposes Restrictions," *Baltimore Sun*, April 18, 2003).

6. When addressing social rather than medical hazards, IRBs are prone to exaggerate risks. On problems social scientists and historians have encountered with IRBs, see Christopher Shea, "Don't Talk to the Humans: The Crackdown on Social Science Research," *Lingua Franca*, September 2000, pp. 27–34; C. K. Gunsalus, "Rethinking Protections for Human Subjects," *Chronicle of Higher Education*, November 15, 2002, p. b24; and American Association of University Professors, "Protecting Human Beings: Institutional Review Boards and Social Science Research," *Academe*, May/June 2001.

7. With localized review boards in place, "new medical technologies continue to move society in totally new directions, with no systematic review of their desirability" (Harold Edger and David J. Rothman, "The Institutional Review Board and Beyond: Future Challenges to the Ethics of Human Experimentation," *Milbank Quarterly* 73, no. 4 [1995]: 499).

8. On the history of the RAC and of its protocol review processes, see Joseph Rainsbury, "Biotechnology on the RAC–FDA/NIH Regulation of Human Gene Therapy," *Food and Drug Law Journal* 55, no. 4 (2000): 575–600.

9. "Wilson said he was only vaguely aware of these experiments, none of which had been published in peer-reviewed journals until after Gelsinger's death. However, the information was widely disseminated in other, less formal ways, such as Web site posting and presentation at scientific meetings" (Deborah Nelson and Rick Weiss, "Hasty Decisions in the Race to a Cure?" *Washington Post*, November 21, 1999).

10. Mulligan noted that two of Wilson's monkeys died after receiving high doses of an adenovirus vector similar to the one later used in the Gelsinger trial. Wilson had concluded, without examining mechanisms leading to the animal fatalities, that lower doses could be safely used in humans. "I was stunned when I found that," Mulligan stated. "If you're searching for a fluke, for some scientific basis for the toxicity seen in the patient who died, with the monkeys you've found it. They died suddenly too. They would have set off my alarms. I'd want to know what killed them and understand it fully before I went into people. Why is giving humans a lesser dose presumed to be safe?" (quoted in Peter Gorner, "Gene Therapy Furor Ends Hemophilia Experiment: Safety Controversy Spurs Reassessment," *Chicago Tribune*, February 8, 2000, p. 1).

11. "Some researchers—such as Art Beaudet of Baylor College of Medicine in Houston and Inder Verma of the Salk Institute in La Jolla, California—say there were warning signs that vectors containing any active adenovirus vector were risky and could cause inflammation. The most dramatic early sign came in a 1993 gene therapy trial conducted by [Ronald] Crystal. He was using an early adenovirus vector to inject healthy genes into the lungs of cystic fibrosis patients. During the experiment, a subject . . . developed a severe inflammatory reaction. . . . Crystal wasn't the only one . . . to report an inflammatory response. Among others, Richard Boucher of the University of North Carolina, Chapel Hill, also ran into the problem in 1994–95 while treating cystic fibrosis patients. He abruptly stopped the trial. . . . Several leaders of the field have said that they knew that directly injecting the livers of volunteers with huge does of immunogenic viral particles (38 trillion at the highest dose)," as specified in the Penn OTC protocol, "was risky. But they did not intervene" (Eliot Marshall, "Gene Therapy on Trial," *Science* 288, no. 5468 [May 12, 2000]: 951–57).

12. Deborah Nelson and Rick Weiss comment on Wilson's success at winning RAC approval of his OTC protocol: "According to several scientists and some NIH committee members, Wilson's charismatic style and his good reputation as a scientist won the day" ("Hasty Decisions in the Race to a Cure?") Discussion of the Penn OTC protocol took place at the RAC meeting of December 4–5, 1995. The NIH Office of Biotechnology Activities holds additional documents bearing on RAC evaluation and approval of the protocol. Written reviews by Robert Erickson and Rochelle Hirschhorn are found in RAC Records, RAC meeting of December 4–5, 1995, tab 1896, pp. 516–22. For an account of the social dynamics—including investigator grandstanding—surrounding evaluation of the first RAC-approved clinical trial, see Jeff Lyon and Peter Gorner, *Altered Fates: Gene Therapy and the Retooling of Human Life* (New York: Norton, 1995).

13. Marshall, "Gene Therapy on Trial," pp. 951–57.

14. On Varmus's views about the RAC and gene-therapy research, see Stolbert, "The Biotech Death of Jesse Gelsinger." On efforts to decommission the RAC, see Rainsbury, "Biotechnology on the RAC–FDA/NIH Regulation of Human Gene Therapy."

15. Philip Noguchi, director of the DCGT described the unit's scientific capabilities in gene therapy at a 1994 meeting of the RAC. According to Noguchi, DCGT protocol-review staff included twenty-four scientists, fourteen Ph.D.'s and ten M.D.'s (or M.D.-Ph.D.'s). See RAC Minutes, September 12–13, 1994, p. 60.

16. Federal administrative law governing FDA disclosures concerning IND exemptions is codified under U.S. 21 CFR 601.51 (d) (1). The FDA commissioner ruled that the outcome in the Penn OTC trial created public interest in disclosure and directed that "summary safety and effectiveness data" from that study be released. That ruling also stated: "The summary information that will be disclosed will be appropriate for public consideration of the issues regarding the safety of OTC gene therapy. Summary information does not include the full reports of investigations required to be submitted for approval, and will not reveal the full administrative record of an IND." See "Disclosure of Information—OTC Gene Therapy," memorandum, dated December 1, 1999, from the commissioner of food and drugs, posted on the CBER Web site (note 3 above provides the URL for access to CBER documents).

17. On variations in the use of advisory committees by the FDA, see Richard A. Rettig, Laurence E. Early, and Richard A. Merrill, eds., *Food and Drug Administration Advisory Committees* (Washington, D.C.: National Academy Press, 1992). For more general commentary on federal scientific advisory boards, see Sheila Jasanoff, *The Fifth Branch: Science Advisors as Policy Makers* (Cambridge: Harvard University Press, 1990); and Bruce L. R. Smith, *The Advisors: Scientists and the Policy Process* (Washington, D.C.: Brookings Institution, 1992).

18. Memo dated March 19, 1996, from Rochelle Hirschhorn to Nelson A. Wivel, director (RAC Records, RAC meeting of December 4–5, 1995, post-meeting correspondence).

19. RAC Minutes, December 4–5, 1995, pp. 46–47.

20. Statement by Batshaw and Wilson from their letter, dated April 25, 1996, to Nelson A. Wivel (RAC Records, RAC meeting of December 4–5, 1995, post-meeting correspondence). Thomas L. Eggerman, FDA staff scientist, gives a different account of Batshaw and Wilson's scientific rationale: "At the pre-IND stage, the FDA raised the question of whether testing this adenovirus vector might be more appropriate in significantly affected male infants who otherwise might die. The sponsors indicated it would be difficult to differentiate between death related to the natural course of the disease and potential adverse events related to vector administration, wanting to study first a relatively healthy population that carried the genetic defect to ascertain an appropriate dose and to characterize the safety profile" (RAC Minutes, December 8–10, 1999, p. 25).

21. Letter, dated April 25, 1996, from Mark. L. Batshaw and James M. Wilson to Nelson A. Wivel (RAC Records, RAC meeting of December 4–5, 1995, post-meeting correspondence).

22. According to Robert Erickson, "Wilson said that you should let people be heroes if they want to be" (quoted in Nelson and Weiss, "Hasty Decisions in the Race to a Cure?"). Penn investigators put considerable effort into securing lay support for their selection of a subject pool. According to Batshaw, the "researchers met with the National Urea Cycle Disorders Foundation (NUCDF), a group of families whose children have OTC deficiency and other urea cycle disorders and with whom the researchers had a prior working relationship. A panel decided unanimously that (1) this study should go forward and (2) it should be conducted in adult, stable individuals who had partial deficiency, because these subjects could give informed consent and because they had metabolic abnormalities in which changes

could be examined following gene transfer" (RAC Minutes, December 8–10, 1999, p. 20). Batshaw arranged for announcements to appear in the NUCDF newsletter and on the organization's Web site saying the Penn researchers were seeking adult volunteers for their study (Nelson and Weiss, "Hasty Decisions in the Race for a Cure?")

23. On the impact since the late 1960s and 1970s of renewed emphasis on rights on policies toward vaccination, and on public health issues more generally, see Deborah A. Stone, "The Resistible Rise of Preventive Medicine," *Health Policy in Transition*, ed. Lawrence D. Brown (Durham: Duke University Press, 1987), pp. 103–28.

24. Paul Root Wolpe, "The Triumph of Autonomy in American Bioethics: A Sociological Perspective," *Bioethics and Society: Constructing the Ethical Enterprise*, ed. Raymond DeVries and Janardan Subedi (Upper Saddle River, N.J.: Prentice-Hall, 1998), p. 47.

25. Julian Savulescu, "Harm, Ethics Committees, and the Gene Therapy Death," *Journal of Medical Ethics* 27, no. 3 (June 2001): 148. On the need for medical practitioners to balance emphasis on patient autonomy with physician beneficence, see Carl E. Schneider, *The Practice of Autonomy: Patients, Doctors, and Medical Decisions* (New York: Oxford University, 1998).

26. Quotation from the transcript of "Talk of the Nation / Science Friday," Ira Flatow, anchor, National Public Radio, January 21, 2002.

27. Quotation from Gorner, "Gene Therapy Furor Ends Hemophilia Experiment," p. 1.

28. Stuart H. Orkin and Arno G. Motulsky, "Report and Recommendations of the Panel to Assess the NIH Investment in Research on Gene Therapy" (National Institutes of Health, December 1995). This document is available at http://www4.od.nih.gov/oba/rac/panelrep.htm.

29. See, for example, Barton J. Bernstein, "The Misguided Quest for the Artificial Heart," *Technology Review* 87, no. 8 (November/December 1984); Diana B. Dutton, *Worse Than the Disease: Pitfalls of Medical Progress* (New York: Cambridge University Press, 1988); and Renée C. Fox and Judith P. Swazey, *Spare Parts: Organ Replacement in American Society* (New York: Oxford University Press, 1992).

30. See the discussion in chapter 1 above.

31. See Warren O. Hagstrom, *The Scientific Community* (New York: Basic, 1965).

32. Richard A. Rettig identifies another trend in the industrialization of biomedical research: pharmaceutical companies' move to outsource clinical trials to contract research organizations. Rettig suggests that these organizations are now competing with academic medical centers for industry-sponsored research. See "The Industrialization of Clinical Research," *Health Affairs* 19, no. 2 (March/April 2000): 129–46.

33. On the commercialization of American universities, see Derek C. Bok, *Universities in the Marketplace: The Commercialization of Higher Education* (Princeton: Princeton University Press, 2003); and Sheldon Krimsky, *Science in the Private Interest: Has the Lure of Profits Corrupted Biomedical Research?* (Lanham, Md.: Rowman & Littlefield, 2003).

34. On biotechnology firms founded by gene-therapy researchers, see Eliot Marshall, "Gene Therapy's Web of Corporate Connections," *Science* 288, no. 5468 (May 12, 2000): 954–55; Paul A. Martin, "Genes as Drugs: The Social Shaping of Gene Therapy and the Reconstruction of Genetic Disease," *Sociology of Health and Illness* 21, no. 5 (1999): 517–38; and Sheryl Gay Stolberg, "Biomedicine Is Receiving New Scrutiny as Scientists Become Entrepreneurs," *New York Times*, February 20, 2000.

35. Scott Hensley, "Targeted Genetics' Genovo Deal Leads to Windfall for Researcher," *Wall Street Journal*, August 10, 2000. For background on Wilson's financial arrangements with Genova and Penn, see Joseph DiStefano, Huntly Collins, and Shankar Vedantam, "Penn Reviewing Gene Institute's Ties to Company," *Philadelphia Inquirer*, February 27, 2000.

36. Gorner, "Gene Therapy Furor Ends Hemophilia Experiment," p. 1

37. See, for example, Theodore Friedmann, "Principles for Human Gene Therapy Studies," *Science* 287, no. 5461 (March 24, 2000): 2163–65.

38. Association of American Medical Colleges, Task Force on Financial Conflicts of Interest, "Protecting Subjects, Preserving Trust, Promotion Progress I: Policy and Guidelines for the Oversight of Individual Financial Conflicts of Interest in Human Subjects Research" and "Protecting Subjects, Preserving Trust, Promotion Progress II: Principles and Recommendations for Oversight of an Institution's Financial Interests in Human Subjects Research," *Academic Medicine* 78, no. 2 (2003): 225–36 and 237–45. A recent report from the Institute of Medicine also recommends conflict-of-interest review. See Daniel D. Federman, Kathi E. Hanna, and Laura L. Rodriquez, eds., Committee on Assessing the System for Protecting Human Research Participants, *Responsible Research: A Systems Approach to Protecting Research Participants* (Washington, D.C.: National Academies Press, 2002).

Selected Bibliography

This bibliography includes selected secondary sources only. See chapter notes for published and unpublished primary sources and additional secondary materials.

Ackerknecht, Erwin H. *Medicine at the Paris Hospital, 1794–1848*. Baltimore: Johns Hopkins University Press, 1967.

Advisory Committee on Human Radiation Experiments. *Final Report*. Washington, D.C.: U.S. Government Printing Office, 1995.

———. *Final Report*. Supplemental vol. 1. Washington, D.C.: U.S. Government Printing Office, 1995.

Altman, Lawrence K. *Who Goes First? The Story of Self-Experimentation in Medicine*. New York: Random House, 1986.

Andrus, E. Cowles, et al., eds. *Advances in Military Medicine*. 2 vols. Boston: Little, Brown, 1948.

Annas, George J., and Michael A. Grodin, eds. *Nazi Doctors and the Nuremberg Code*. New York: Oxford University Press, 1992.

Anspach, Renée R. *Deciding Who Lives: Fateful Choices in the Intensive-Care Nursery*. Berkeley and Los Angeles: University of California Press, 1993.

Baker, Robert, ed. *The Codification of Medical Morality*. Vol. 2, *Anglo-American Medical Ethics and Medicine Jurisprudence in the Nineteenth Century*. Dordrecht: Kluwer, 1995.

Baker, Robert, Dorothy Porter, and Roy Porter, eds. *The Codification of Medical Morality*. Vol. 1, *Medical Ethics and Etiquette in the Eighteenth Century*. Dordrecht: Kluwer, 1993.

Baldwin, Peter. *Contagion and the State in Europe, 1830–1930*. Cambridge: Cambridge University Press, 1999.

Barber, Bernard, et al. *Research on Human Subjects: Problems of Social Control in Medical Experimentation*. New Brunswick: Transaction Books, 1979.

Baxby, Derrick. *Jenner's Smallpox Vaccine*. London: Heinemann, 1981.

Beauchamp, Tom L., and James F. Childress. *Principles of Biomedical Ethics*. New York: Oxford University Press, 1983.

Beck, Ann. "Issues in the Anti-Vaccination Movement in England." *Medical History* 4, no. 4 (October 1960): 310–21.

Beck, Ulrich. *Risk Society: Toward a New Modernity*. Trans. Mark Ritter. London: Sage, 1992.

Beecher, Henry K. "Ethics and Clinical Research." *New England Journal of Medicine* 74 (1966): 1354–60.

Ben-David, Joseph. "Scientific Productivity and Academic Organization in Nineteenth Century Medicine." *American Sociological Review* 25, no. 6 (1960): 828–43.

Benison, Saul. "History of Polio Research in the United States: Appraisal and Lessons." In *The Twentieth-Century Sciences*, ed. Gerald Holton, pp. 308–43. New York: Norton, 1970.

———. "In Defense of Medical Research." *Harvard Medical Alumni Bulletin* 44, no. 3 (1970): 16–23.

———. "Poliomyelitis and the Rockefeller Institute: Social Effects and Institutional Response." *Journal of the History of Medicine* 29, no. 1 (January 1974): 74–92.

———. "Speculation and Experimentation in Early Poliomyelitis Research." *Clio Medica* 10 (1975): 1–22.

———. *Tom Rivers: Reflections on a Life in Medicine and Science*. Cambridge: MIT Press, 1967.

Berk, Lawrence, B. "Polio Vaccine Trials of 1935." *Transactions of the College of Physicians of Philadelphia*, ser. 5, 11, no. 4 (1989): 321–336.

Bernstein, Barton J. "The Misguided Quest for the Artificial Heart." *Technology Review* 87, no. 8 (November/December 1984): 12.

Bok, Derek C. *Universities in the Marketplace: The Commercialization of Higher Education*. Princeton: Princeton University Press, 2003.

Bosk, Charles L. *All God's Mistakes: Genetic Counseling in a Pediatric Hospital*. Chicago: University of Chicago Press, 1992.

———. *Forgive and Remember: Managing Medical Failure*. Chicago: University of Chicago Press, 1979.

———. "Social Control and Physicians: The Oscillation of Cynicism and Idealism in Sociological Theory." In *Social Controls in the Medical Profession*, ed. Judith Swazey and Stephen Scher, pp. 31–51. Boston: Oelgeschlager, Gunn & Hain, 1985.

Boston University, Law-Medicine Research Institute. "Summary Report of Two Questionnaire Surveys," *Final Report of Administrative Practices in Clinical Research*. Boston: Law-Medicine Research Institute, Boston University, 1963.

Brandt, Allan M. "Polio, Politics, Publicity, and Duplicity: Ethical Aspects in the Development of the Salk Vaccine." *International Journal of Health Services* 8, no. 2 (1978): 257–70.

Brock, Dan W. "Public Policy and Bioethics." In *Encyclopedia of Bioethics*, ed. Warren T. Reich, 4:2181–87. New York: Free Press, 1995.

Brock, Thomas D. *Robert Koch*. Madison: Science Tech, 1988.

Bucchi, Massimiano. "The Public Science of Louis Pasteur: The Experiment on Anthrax

Vaccine in the Popular Press of the Time." *History and Philosophy of the Life Sciences* 19 (1997): 181–209.

Cady, Elwyn L. Jr. "Medical Malpractice: What about Experimentation?" *Annals of Western Medicine and Surgery* 6 (1952): 164–70.

Calhoun, Craig, and Henry K. Hiller. "Coping with Insidious Injuries: The Case of Johns-Manville Corporation and Asbestos Exposure." *Social Problems* 35, no. 2 (April 1988): 162–81.

Carruthers, Bruce G., and Terence C. Halliday. *Rescuing Business: The Making of Corporate Bankruptcy Law in England and the United States.* Oxford: Clarendon Press, 1998.

Carter, Richard. *Breakthrough: The Saga of Jonas Salk.* New York: Trident, 1966.

Chambliss, Daniel F. *Beyond Caring: Hospitals, Nurses, and the Social Organization of Ethics.* Chicago: University of Chicago Press, 1996.

———. Is Bioethics Irrelevant? *Contemporary Sociology* 22, no. 5 (1993): 649–52.

Chase, Allan. *Magic Shots.* New York: William Morrow, 1982.

Cheit, Ross E. *Setting Safety Standards: Regulation in the Public and Private Sectors.* Berkeley and Los Angeles: University of California Press, 1990.

Clarke, Adele E. "Research Materials and Reproductive Science in the United States, 1910–1940." In *Physiology in the American Context, 1985–1940,* ed. Gerald Geison, pp. 323–50. Bethesda: American Philosophical Society, 1987.

Clarke, Lee. "The Disqualification Heuristic: When Do Organizations Misperceive Risk?" *Research on Social Problems and Public Policy* 5 (1993): 289–312.

———. "Explaining Choices among Technological Risks." *Social Problems* 35, no. 1 (1988): 22–35.

———. *Mission Improbable: Using Fantasy Documents to Tame Disaster.* Chicago: University of Chicago Press, 1999.

Clarke, Lee, and James F. Short. "Social Organization and Risk: Some Current Controversies." *Annual Review of Sociology* 19 (1993): 375–99.

Collins, Harry M. "The TEA Set: Tacit Knowledge and Scientific Networks." *Science Studies* 4 (1974): 165–86.

Cochrane, Rexmond C. *The National Academy of Science: The First Hundred Years, 1863–1963.* Washington D.C.: National Academy of Sciences, 1978.

Corner, George W. *A History of the Rockefeller Institute.* New York: Rockefeller Institute Press, 1964.

Crane, Diana. *The Sanctity of Life.* New York: Russell Sage, 1975.

Curran, William C. "Government Regulation of the Use of Human Subjects in Medical Research: The Approach of Two Federal Agencies." In *Experimentation with Human Subjects,* ed. Paul A. Freund, pp. 402–53. New York: George Braziller, 1970.

Cushing, Harvey. *The Life of Sir William Osler.* Vol. 2. Oxford: Clarendon Press, 1925.

Daston, Lorraine. *Classical Probability in the Enlightenment.* Princeton: Princeton University Press, 1988.

Dietz, Thomas. M., and Robert W. Rycroft. *The Risk Professionals.* New York: Sage, 1987.

DeVries, Raymond, and Janardan Subedi, eds. *Bioethics and Society: Constructing the Ethical Enterprise.* Upper Saddle River, N.J.: Prentice-Hall, 1998.

DiMaggio, Paul J. "Constructing an Organizational Field as a Professional Project: U.S. Art Museums, 1920–1940." In *New Institutionalism in Organizational Analysis*, ed. Walter W. Powell and Paul J. DiMaggio, pp. 267–92. Chicago: University of Chicago Press, 1991.

DiMaggio, Paul J., and Walter W. Powell. "The Iron Cage Revisited: Institutional Isomorphism and Collective Rationality." *American Sociological Review* 48 (1983): 147–60.

Dixon, C. W. *Smallpox*. London: Churchill, 1962.

Dobbin, Frank R., Lauren B. Edelman, John W. Meyer, and W. Richard Scott. "Equal Opportunity Law and the Construction of Internal Labor Markets." *American Journal of Sociology* 99 (1993): 396–427

Douglas, Mary. *Risk Acceptability according to the Social Sciences*. New York: Russell Sage, 1985.

Douglas, Mary, and Aaron Wildavsky. *Risk and Culture*. Berkeley and Los Angeles: University of California Press, 1982.

Draper, Elaine. "Preventive Law by Corporate Professional Team Players: Liability and Responsibility in the Work of Company Doctors." *Journal of Contemporary Health Law and Policy* 15 (1999): 525–607.

Dubos, René J. *Louis Pasteur: Free Lance of Science*. New York: Charles Schribner, 1976.

Durkheim, Emile. *Division of Labor in Society*. Trans. George Simpson. 1893. New York: Free Press, 1964.

Dutton, Diana B. *Worse Than the Disease: Pitfalls of Medical Progress*. New York: Cambridge University Press, 1988.

Edelman, Lauren B. "Legal Ambiguity and Symbolic Structures: Organizational Mediation of Law." *American Journal of Sociology* 97 (1992): 1530–76.

———. "Legal Environments and Organizational Governance: The Expansion of Due Process in the American Workplace." *American Journal of Sociology* 95 (1990): 1401–40.

Edelman, Lauren B., Steven E. Abraham, and Howard S. Erlanger. "Professional Construction of Law: The Inflated Threat of Wrongful Discharge." *Law and Society Review* 25, no. 1 (1992): 47–83.

Edelman, Lauren B., and Mark C. Suchman. "The Legal Environment of Organizations." *Annual Review of Sociology* 23 (1997): 479–515.

Edelman, Lauren B., Christopher Uggen, and Howard S. Erlanger. "The Endogeneity of Legal Regulation: Grievance Procedures as Rational Myth." *American Journal of Sociology* 105 (1999): 406–54.

Edger, Harold, and David J. Rothman. "The Institutional Review Board and Beyond: Future Challenges to the Ethics of Human Experimentation." *Milbank Quarterly* 73, no. 4 (1995): 489–506.

Epstein, Steven. *Impure Science: AIDS, Activism, and the Politics of Knowledge*. Berkeley and Los Angeles: University of California Press, 1996.

Erikson, Kai. *Wayward Puritans: A Study in the Sociology of Deviance*. New York: Wiley, 1966.

Evans, John H. *Playing God: Human Genetic Engineering and the Rationalization of Public Bioethical Debate*. Chicago: University of Chicago Press, 2002.

Faden, Ruth R., and Tom L. Beauchamp. *A History and Theory of Informed Consent*. New York: Oxford University Press, 1986.

Farley, John. *To Cast Out Disease: A History of the International Health Division of Rockefeller Foundation, 1913–1951.* Oxford: Oxford University Press, 2004.

Fletcher, Joseph. "Our Shameful Waste of Human Tissue: An Ethical Problem for the Living and the Dead." In *The Religious Situation, 1969,* ed. Donald R. Cutler, pp. 223–52. Boston: Beacon Press, 1969.

Fosdick, Raymond B. *The Story of the Rockefeller Foundation.* New York: Harper, 1952.

Fox, Renée C. "The Evolution of American Bioethics: A Sociological Perspective." In *Social Science Perspectives on Medical Ethics,* ed. George Weisz, pp. 201–17. Dordrecht: Kluwer, 1990.

———. "The Evolution of Medical Uncertainty." *Milbank Memorial Fund Quarterly* 58, no. 1 (1980): 1–49.

———. *Experiment Perilous.* Glencoe, Ill.: Free Press, 1959.

———. "The Sociology of Bioethics" In *The Sociology of Medicine: A Participant Observer's View,* pp. 224–76. Englewood Cliffs, N.J.: Prentice-Hall, 1989.

———. "Training for Uncertainty." In *The Student Physician,* ed. Robert K. Merton, George G. Reader, and Patricia L. Kendall, pp. 207–41. Cambridge: Harvard University Press, 1957.

Fox, Renée C., and Judith P. Swazey. *Courage to Fail: A Social View of Organ Transplants and Dialysis.* 1974. Chicago: University of Chicago Press, 1978.

———. "Medical Morality Is Not Bioethics: Medical Ethics in China and the United States." *Perspectives in Biology and Medicine* 27, no. 3 (spring 1984): 336–60.

———. *Spare Parts: Organ Replacement in American Society.* New York: Oxford University Press, 1992.

Frankel, Mark S. "The Development of Policy Guidelines Governing Human Experimentation in the United States: A Case Study of Public Policy-Making for Science and Technology." *Ethics in Science and Medicine* 2 (1975): 43–59.

———. *The Public Health Service Guidelines Governing Research Involving Human Subjects: An Analysis of the Policy Making Process.* Program of Policy Studies in Science and Technology, Monograph no. 10. Washington, D.C.: George Washington University, 1972.

———. "Public Policy Making for Biomedical Research: The Case of Human Experimentation." Ph.D. diss., George Washington University, 1976.

Freidson, Eliot. *Doctoring Together.* New York: Elsevier, 1975.

———. *Profession of Medicine.* New York: Harper and Row, 1970.

French, Richard D. *Antivivisection and Medical Science in Victorian Society.* Princeton: Princeton University Press, 1975.

Freudenburg, William R. "Risk and Recreancy: Weber, the Division of Labor, and the Rationality of Risk Perception," *Social Forces* 71, no. 4 (June 1993): 909–32.

Freund, Paul A., ed. *Experimentation with Human Subjects.* New York: George Braziller, 1970.

Friedmann, Theodore. "Principles for Human Gene Therapy Studies." *Science* 287, no. 5461 (March 24, 2000): 2163–65.

Gunsalus, C. K. "Rethinking Protections for Human Subjects." *Chronicle of Higher Education,* November 15, 2002, p. b24.

Galambos, Louis, and Jane Eliot Sewell. *Networks of Innovation: Vaccine Development at Merck, Sharp and Dohme, and Mulford, 1895–1995*. Cambridge: Cambridge University Press, 1995.

Geertz, Clifford. *Local Knowledge*. New York: Basic Books, 1983.

Geison, Gerald L. "Divided We Stand: Physiologists and Clinicians in the American Context." In *The Therapeutic Revolutions: Essays in the Social History of American Medicine*, ed. Morris J. Vogel and Charles E. Rosenberg, pp. 67–90. Philadelphia: University of Pennsylvania, 1977.

———. "Pasteur's Work on Rabies: Reexamining the Ethical Issues. *Hastings Center Report* 8, no. 2 (1978): 26–33.

———. *The Private Science of Louis Pasteur*. Princeton: Princeton University Press, 1995.

Gieryn, Thomas F. "Boundary-Work and the Demarcation of Science from Non-Science: Strains and Interests in Professional Ideologies of Scientists." *American Sociological Review* 48 (December 1983): 781–95.

———. *Cultural Boundaries of Science: Credibility on the Line*. Chicago: University of Chicago Press, 1999.

Gilbert, G. Nigel. "The Transformation of Research Findings into Scientific Knowledge." *Social Studies of Science* 6 (1976): 281–306.

Golinski, Jan. *Science as Public Culture: Chemistry and Enlightenment in Britain, 1760–1820*. New York: Cambridge University Press, 1992.

Goode, William. Community within a Community: The Professions." *American Sociological Review* 22 (1957): 194–200.

Grafton, Thurman S. "The Founding and Early History of the National Society for Medical Research." *Laboratory Animal Science* 30, no. 4 (August 1980): 759–64.

Gray, Bradford H. "Bioethics Commissions: What Can We Learn from Past Successes and Failures?" In *Society's Choices: Social and Ethical Decision Making in Biomedicine*, ed. Ruth E. Bulger, Elizabeth M. Bobby, and Harvey V. Fineberg, pp. 261–306. Washington D.C.: National Academy Press, 1995.

Griffith, Belver C., and Nicholas C. Mullins. "Coherent Social Groups in Scientific Change." *Science* 117 (1972): 959–64.

Grimshaw, Margaret L. "Scientific Specialization and the Poliovirus Controversy in the Years before World War II." *Bulletin of the History of Medicine* 69, no. 1 (spring 1995): 44–65.

Haber, Samuel. "The Professions and Higher Education in America: A Historical View." In *Higher Education and the Labor Market*, ed. Margaret S. Gordon. New York: Carnegie Foundation, 1974.

Hacking, Ian. *The Emergence of Probability*. London: Cambridge University Press, 1975.

Hagstrom, Warren O. *The Scientific Community*. New York: Basic Books, 1965.

Halpern, Sydney A. "Constructing Moral Boundaries: Public Discourse on Human Experimentation in Twentieth-Century America." In *Bioethics in Social Context*, ed. Barry C. Hoffmaster, pp. 69–89. Philadelphia: Temple University Press, 2000.

———. "Medical Authority and the Culture of Rights." *Journal of Health Politics, Policy, and Law* 29, nos. 4–5 (2004).

———. "Professional Schools in the American University: The Evolving Dilemma of Research and Practice." In *The Academic Profession: National, Disciplinary, and Institutional Settings,* ed. Burton R. Clark, pp. 304–30. Berkeley and Los Angeles: University of California Press, 1987.

Hammonds, Evelynn M. *Childhood's Deadly Scourge: The Campaign to Control Diphtheria in New York City, 1880–1930.* Baltimore: Johns Hopkins University Press, 1999.

Hansen, Bert. "America's First Medical Breakthrough: How Popular Excitement about French Rabies Cure in 1885 Raised New Expectations for Medical Progress." *American Historical Review* 103 (April 1998): 373–418.

———. "New Images of a New Medicine: Visual Evidence for the Widespread Popularity of Therapeutic Discoveries in America after 1885." *Bulletin of the History of Medicine* 73, no. 4 (winter 1999): 679–84.

Hardy, Anne. *Epidemic Streets: Infectious Disease and the Rise of Preventive Medicine, 1856–1900.* Oxford: Clarendon Press, 1993.

———. "Liberty, Equality, and Immunization: The English Experience since 1800." Paper delivered at the meetings of the American Association for the History of Medicine, Boston, May 2003.

Harkness, Jon H. "Research behind Bars: A History of Nontherapeutic Research on American Prisoners." Ph.D. diss., University of Wisconsin, Madison, 1996.

Haskins, Thomas L. *Jean d'Alembert: Science and the Enlightenment.* Oxford: Clarendon Press, 1970.

Havighurst, Clarke C. "The Place of Private Accreditation among the Instruments of Government." *Law and Contemporary Problems* 57, no. 4 (1995): 1–14.

Heimer, Carol A. "Explaining Variation in the Impact of the Law: Organizations, Institutions, and Professions. *Studies in Law, Politics, and Society* 15 (1996): 29–59.

———. "Insuring More, Ensuring Less: The Costs and Benefits of Private Regulation through Insurance." In *Embracing Risk,* ed. Tom Backer and Jonathan Simon. Chicago: University of Chicago Press, 2002.

———. *Reactive Risk and Rational Action: Managing Moral Hazard in Insurance Contracts.* Berkeley and Los Angeles: University of California Press, 1985.

Heimer, Carol A., and Lisa R. Staffen. *For the Sake of the Children: The Social Organization of Responsibility in the Hospital and the Home.* Chicago: University of Chicago Press, 1998.

Hilgartner, Stephen, and Charles L. Bosk. "The Rise and Fall of Social Problems: A Public Arenas Model." *American Journal of Sociology* 94, no. 1 (July 1988): 53–78.

Hill, Austin Bradford. "Medical Ethics and Controlled Clinical Trials." In *Clinical Investigation in Medicine: Legal, Ethical, and Moral Aspects,* ed. Irving Ladimer and Roger Newman, pp. 370–83. Boston: Boston University Law-Medicine Research Institute, 1963.

Hinchliffe, Joseph J. "Anticipatory Democracy: The Influence of the Imagined Public on Safety Regulation." Ph.D. diss., University of Illinois at Urbana-Champaign, 2002.

Hoffmaster, Barry C., ed. *Bioethics in Social Context.* Philadelphia: Temple University Press, 2001.

Hollinger, David A. "Inquiry and Uplift: Late Nineteenth Century American Academics and the Moral Efficiency of Scientific Practice." In *The Authority of Experts: Studies in*

History and Theory, ed. Thomas L. Haskell, pp. 142–56. Bloomington: Indiana University Press, 1984.

Horstmann, Dorothy. "The Poliomyelitis Story: A Scientific Hegira." *Yale Journal of Biology and Medicine* 58 (1985): 79–90.

Jasanoff, Sheila. *The Fifth Branch: Science Advisors as Policy Makers.* Cambridge: Harvard University Press, 1990.

———. *Risk Management and Political Culture.* New York: Russell Sage, 1986.

Jonsen, Albert R. *The Birth of Bioethics.* New York: Oxford University Press, 1998.

Jonsen, Albert R., and Andrew Jameton. "History of Medical Ethics: The United States in the Twentieth Century." *Encyclopedia of Bioethics,* ed. Warren T. Reich, 3: 1616–32. New York: Free Press, 1995.

Katz, Jay. *The Silent World of Doctor and Patient.* New York: Free Press, 1984.

Kaufman, Martin. "The American Anti-Vaccinationists and Their Arguments." *Bulletin of the History of Medicine* 41 (1967): 463–79.

Keefer, Chester S. "Dr. Richards as Chairman of the Committee on Medical Research." *Annals of Internal Medicine* 71, no. 5 (November 1969), S8:61–70.

Kitch, Edward W., Geoffrey Evans, and Robyn Gopin. "U. S. Law." In *Vaccines,* eds. Stanley A. Plotkin and Walter A. Orenstein, pp. 1165–86. Philadelphia: Saunders, 1999.

Klein, Aaron E. *Trial by Fury: The Polio Vaccine Controversy.* New York: Scribner's, 1972.

Kramer, Victor H. *The National Institute of Health: A Study in Public Administration.* New Haven: Quinnipiack, 1937.

Krimsky, Sheldon. *Science in the Private Interest: Has the Lure of Profits Corrupted Biomedical Research?* Lanham, Md.: Rowman & Littlefield, 2003.

Ladimer, Irving. "Law and Medicine, a Symposium: Ethical and Legal Aspects of Medical Research on Human Beings." *Journal of Public Law* 3, no. 1 (spring 1954): 466–511.

LaFollette, Marcel C. *Making Science Our Own: Public Images of Science, 1910–1955.* Chicago: University of Chicago Press, 1990.

Lamont, Michèle, and Virag Molnar. "The Study of Boundaries in the Social Sciences." *Annual Review of Sociology* 28 (August 2002): 157–95.

Larson, Magali Sarfatti. *The Rise of Professionalism: A Sociological Analysis.* Berkeley and Los Angeles: University of California Press, 1977.

Laumann, Edward O., and David Knoke. *The Organizational State: Social Choice in National Policy Domains.* Madison: University of Wisconsin Press, 1987.

Lederer, Susan E. "The Controversy over Animal Experimentation in America, 1880–1914." In *Vivisection in Historical Perspective,* ed. Nicolaas A. Rupke, pp. 236–58. London: Routledge, 1987.

———. "Hideyo Noguchi's Luetin Experiment and the Antivivisectionists." *Isis* 76 (1985): 31–48.

———. "Political Animals: The Shaping of Biomedical Research Literature in Twentieth-Century America." *Isis* 83, no. 1 (1992): 61–79.

———. *Subjected to Science: Human Experimentation in America before the Second World War.* Baltimore: Johns Hopkins University Press, 1995.

Levine, Robert J. "Ethical Practices, Institutional Oversight, and Enforcement. "In *Interna-*

tional Encyclopedia of the Social and Behavioral Sciences, ed. Neil J. Smelser and P. B. Baltes, pp. 4770–74. New York: Elsevier, 2001.

———. *Ethics and Regulation of Clinical Research*. Baltimore: Urban & Schwarzenberg, 1986.

Liebenau, Jonathan. *Medical Science and Medical Industry: The Formation of the American Pharmaceutical Industry*. Baltimore: Johns Hopkins University Press, 1987.

Light, Donald. "Uncertainty and Control in Professional Training." *Journal of Health and Social Behavior* 6 (1979): 141–51.

Ludmerer, Kenneth M. *Learning to Heal: The Development of American Medical Education*. New York: Basic Books, 1985.

Luhmann, Niklas. *Risk: A Sociological Theory*. Trans. Rhodes Barrett. New York: Aldine de Gruyter, 1993.

Lupton, Deborah. *Risk*. London: Routledge, 2003.

Lyon, Jeff, and Peter Gorner. *Altered Fates: Gene Therapy and the Retooling of Human Life*. New York: Norton, 1995.

MacLeod, R. M. "Law, Medicine, and Public Opinion: The Resistance to Compulsory Health Legislation, 1870–1907. *Public Law*, summer 1967, pp. 107–28, and autumn 1967, pp. 189–210.

Mahoney, Tom. *The Merchants of Life: An Account of the American Pharmaceutical Industry*. New York: Harper, 1959.

Mariner, Wendy. "Informed Consent in the Post-Modern Era." *Law and Social Inquiry* 13, no. 2 (1988): 385–406.

Marks, Harry M. "Local Knowledge: Experimental Communities and Experimental Practices, 1918–1950." Paper delivered at the Conference on Twentieth Century Health Science, University of California, San Francisco, May 1988.

———. "Notes from the Underground: The Social Organization of Therapeutic Research." In *Grand Rounds: One Hundred Years of Internal Medicine*, ed. Russell C. Maulitz and Diana E. Long, pp. 297–336. Philadelphia: University of Pennsylvania Press, 1988.

———. *The Progress of Experiment: Science and Therapeutic Reform in the United States, 1900–1990*. Cambridge: Cambridge University Press, 1997.

———. "Where Do Ethics Come From? The Case of Human Experimentation." Paper delivered at the Center for Biomedical Ethics, Case Western Reserve University, March 1988.

———. "Where Do Ethics Come From? The Role of Disciplines and Institutions." Paper delivered at the Conference on Ethical Issues in Clinical Trials, University of Alabama at Birmingham, February 25–26, 2000.

Marshall, Eliot. "Gene Therapy on Trial." *Science* 288, no. 5468 (May 12, 2000): 951–57.

Matthews, J. Rosser. *Quantification and the Quest for Medical Certainty*. Princeton: Princeton University Press, 1999.

Martin, Paul A. "Genes as Drugs: The Social Shaping of Gene Therapy and the Reconstruction of Genetic Disease." *Sociology of Health and Illness* 21, no. 5 (1999): 517–38.

McCann, Diane J., and John R. Pettit. "A Report on Adverse Effects of Insurance for Human Subjects." In *Compensating for Research Injuries*, vol. 2, *Appendices*, pp. 239–71.

President's Commission for the Study of Ethical Problems in Medical and Biomedical and Behavioral Research. Washington D.C.: U.S. Government Printing Office, 1982.

McCoid, Allan H. "A Reappraisal of Liability for Unauthorized Medical Treatment." *Minnesota Law Review* 41, no. 4 (March 1957): 381–434.

McNeill, Paul M. *The Ethics and Politics of Human Experimentation.* Cambridge: Cambridge University Press, 1993.

Meldrum, Marcia L. "The Historical Feud over Polio Vaccine: How Could a Killed Vaccine Contain a Natural Disease?" *Western Journal of Medicine* 171 (October 1999): 271–73.

Merton, Robert K. "The Normative Structure of Science." 1942. In *The Sociology of Science,* ed. Normal W. Storer, pp. 267–85. Chicago: University of Chicago Press, 1973.

———. "Science and the Social Order." 1938. In *The Sociology of Science,* ed. Normal W. Storer, pp. 254–66. Chicago: University of Chicago Press, 1973.

Meyer, John W., and Brian Rowan. "Institutionalized Organizations: Formal Structure as Myth and Ceremony." *American Journal of Sociology* 83 (1977): 340–63.

Meyer, John W., and W. Richard Scott, eds. *Organizational Environments: Ritual and Rationality.* 1983. Newbury Park, Calif.: Sage, 1992.

Miller, Genevieve. *Adoption of Inoculation of Smallpox in England and France.* Philadelphia: University of Pennsylvania Press, 1957.

Miller, Genevieve. "Smallpox Inoculation in England and America: A Reappraisal." *William and Mary Quarterly,* ser. 3, 13, no. 4 (October 1956): 476–92.

Moore, Francis D. "Therapeutic Innovation: Ethical Boundaries in the Initial Clinical Trials of New Drugs and Surgical Procedures." In *Experimentation with Human Subjects,* ed. Paul A. Freund, pp. 358–82. New York: George Braziller, 1970.

Moore, Kelly. "Organizing Integrity: American Science and the Creation of Public Interest Organizations." *American Journal of Sociology* 101, no. 6 (1996): 1592–1627.

Moreno, Jonathan D. *Undue Risk: Secret State Experiments on Humans.* New York: W. H. Freeman, 1999.

Moulin, Anne Marie. "Le Métaphore vaccine: De l'inoculation à la vaccinologie." *History and Philosophy of Life Science* 14 (1992): 271–97.

Mulkay, Michael J. "Some Aspects of Cultural Growth in the Natural Sciences." *Social Research* 36 (1969): 22–52.

Mulkay, Michael J., G. Nigel Gilbert, and Steve Woolgar. "Problem Areas and Research Networks in Science." *Sociology* 9 (1975): 187–203.

National Commission for the Protection of Human Subjects of Biomedical and Behavioral Research. *The Belmont Report: Ethical Principles and Guidelines for the Protection of Human Subjects.* Washington, D.C.: U.S. Government Printing Office, 1978.

Nelkin, Dorothy. *Selling Science.* New York: W. H. Freeman, 1995.

———. "Social Controls in the Changing Context of Science." In *Social Controls in the Medical Profession,* ed. Judith Swazey and Stephen Scher, pp. 83–94. Boston: Oelgeschlager, Gunn and Hain, 1985.

Osler, William. "The Influence of Louis on American Medicine." In *An Alabama Student, and Other Biographical Essays,* pp. 189–210. New York: Oxford University Press, 1908.

Parkman, Paul D., and M. Carolyn Hardegree. "Regulation and the Testing of Vaccines." In

Vaccines, ed. Stanley A. Plotkin and Walter A. Orenstein, pp. 1131–43. Philadelphia: Saunders, 1999.

Parish, H. J. *History of Immunization.* London: Livingstone, 1965.

Paul, John R. *A History of Poliomyelitis.* New Haven: Yale University Press, 1971.

Pernick, Martin. S. "The Patient's Role in Medical Decisionmaking: A Social History of Informed Consent in Medical Therapy." In *Making Health Care Decisions,* ed. President's Commission for the Study of Ethical Problems in Medicine and Biomedical and Behavioral Research, 3:1–35. Washington, D.C.: U.S. Government Printing Office, 1982.

Pernick, Martin S. *A Calculus of Suffering: Pain, Professionalism, and Anesthesia in Nineteenth Century America.* New York: Columbia University Press, 1985.

Pittman, Margaret. "The Regulation of Biologic Products, 1902–1972." In *National Institute of Allergy and Infectious Disease: Intramural Contributions, 1887–1987,* ed. Harriet R. Greenwald and Victoria A. Harden, pp. 61–70. Washington, D.C.: National Institutes of Health, 1987.

Plotkin, Stanley A., and Susan L. Plotkin. "Vaccination: One Hundred Years Later." In *World's Debt to Pasteur,* ed. Hilary Koprowsky and Stanley A. Plotkin, pp. 83–106. Wistar Symposium Series 3. New York: Liss, 1985.

Plotkin, Susan L., and Stanley A. Plotkin. "A Short History of Vaccination." In *Vaccines,* ed. Stanley A. Plotkin and Walter A. Orenstein, pp. 1–12. Philadelphia: Saunders, 1999.

Porter, Dorothy, and Roy Porter. "The Politics of Prevention: Anti-Vaccination and Public Health in Nineteenth Century England. *Medical History* 32, no. 3 (July 1988): 231–52.

Porter, Theodore M. *Trust in Numbers: The Pursuit of Objectivity in Science and Public Life.* Princeton: Princeton University Press, 1995.

Powell, Walter W., and Paul J. DiMaggio, eds. *New Institutionalism in Organizational Analysis.* Chicago: University of Chicago Press, 1991.

President's Commission for the Study of Ethical Problems in Medical and Biomedical and Behavioral Research. *Compensating for Research Injuries.* Vol. 1, *Report.* Vol. 2, *Appendices.* Washington D.C.: U.S. Government Printing Office, 1982.

Rainsbury, Joseph M. "Biotechnology on the RAC–FDA/NIH Regulation of Human Gene Therapy." *Food and Drug Law Journal* 55, no. 4 (2000): 576–600.

Razell, Peter. *The Conquest of Smallpox: The Impact of Inoculation on Smallpox in Eighteenth Century Britain.* Sussex: Caliban Books, 1977.

Rees, Joseph V. *Hostages of Each Other: The Transformation of Nuclear Safety since Three Mile Island.* Chicago: University of Chicago Press, 1994.

Reiser, Stanley Joel, Arthur J. Dyck, and William J. Curran, eds. *Ethics in Medicine: Historical Perspectives and Contemporary Concerns.* Cambridge: MIT Press, 1977.

Rettig, Richard A. "The Industrialization of Clinical Research," *Health Affairs* 19, no. 2 (March/April 2000): 129–46.

Rettig, Richard A., Laurence E. Early, and Richard A. Merrill, eds. *Food and Drug Administration Advisory Committees.* Washington, D.C.: National Academy Press, 1992.

Rivers, Thomas M. "The Story of Research on Poliomyelitis." *Proceedings of the American Philosophical Society* 98, no. 4 (August 1954): 250–54.

Robbins, Frederick C. "The History of Polio Vaccine Development." In *Vaccines*, ed. Stanley A. Plotkin and Walter A. Orenstein, pp. 13–27. Philadelphia: Saunders, 1999.

Rogers, Naomi. *Dirt and Disease: Polio before FDR*. New Brunswick: Rutgers University Press, 1992.

Rosenberg, Charles E. "The Therapeutic Revolution: Medicine, Meaning, and Social Change in Nineteenth Century America. *Perspectives in Biology and Medicine* 20 (summer 1977): 485–506.

Rothman, David J. "Human Experimentation and the Origins of Bioethics in the United States." In *Social Science Perspectives on Medical Ethics*, ed. George Weisz, pp. 185–200. Dordrecht: Kluwer, 1990.

———. *Strangers at the Bedside: A History of How Law and Bioethics Transformed Medical Decision Making*. New York: Basic Books, 1991.

Rupke, Nicolaas A., ed. *Vivisection in Historical Perspective*. London: Routledge, 1990.

Rusnock, Andrea A. *Vital Accounts: Quantifying Health and Population in Eighteenth-Century England and France*. Cambridge: Cambridge University Press, 2002.

———. "The Weight of Evidence and the Burden of Authority: Case Histories, Medical Statistics, and Smallpox Inoculation." In *Medicine in the Enlightenment*, ed. Roy Porter, pp. 289–315. Wellcome Institute Series in the History of Medicine 29. Amsterdam: Rodopi, 1995.

Rutstein, David D. "The Ethical Design of Human Experiments." In *Experimentation with Human Subjects* ed. Paul A. Freund, pp. 383–401. New York: George Braziller, 1970.

Sanders, Joseph. "Firm Risk Management in the Face of Product Liability Rules." In *Organizations, Uncertainty, and Risk*, ed. James F. Short Jr. and Lee Clarke, pp. 57–81. Boulder: Westview Press, 1992.

Savulescu, Julian. "Harm, Ethics Committees, and the Gene Therapy Death." *Journal of Medical Ethics* 27, no. 3 (June 2001): 148–50.

Schaffner, Kenneth F. "Ethical Problems in Clinical Trials." *Journal of Medicine and Philosophy* 11 (1986): 297–315.

Schneider, Carl E. *The Practice of Autonomy: Patients, Doctors, and Medical Decisions*. New York: Oxford University Press, 1998.

Scott, Colin. "Private Regulation of the Public Sector: A Neglected Facet of Contemporary Governance." *Journal of Law and Society* 29, no. 1 (2002): 56–76.

Scott, W. Richard. *Organizations: Rational, Natural, and Open Systems*. 4th ed. Englewood Cliffs, N.J.: Prentice-Hall, 1998.

Scott, W. Richard, and John W. Meyer. "The Organization of Societal Sectors: Propositions and Early Evidence." In *New Institutionalism in Organizational Analysis*, ed. Walter W. Powell and Paul J. DiMaggio, pp. 108–40. Chicago: University of Chicago Press, 1991.

Shannon, James A. "The Advancement of Medical Research: A Twenty-Year View of the Role of the National Institutes of Health." *Journal of Medical Education* 42, no. 2 (February 1967): 97–108.

Shapin, Steven. "Pump and Circumstance: Robert Boyle's Literary Technology." *Social Studies of Science* 14 (1984): 481–520.

Shapin, Steven, and Simon Schaffer. *Leviathan and the Air-Pump: Hobbes, Boyle, and the Experimental Life*. Princeton: Princeton University Press, 1985.

Shapiro, Barbara J. *Probability and Certainty in Seventeenth Century Britain.* Princeton: Princeton University Press, 1983.

Shea, Christopher. "Don't Talk to the Humans: The Crackdown on Social Science Research." *Lingua Franca,* September 2000, pp. 27–34.

Short, James F. Jr. "The Social Fabric at Risk: Toward the Social Transformation of Risk Analysis," *American Sociological Review* 49 (1984): 711–25.

Short, James F. Jr., and Lee Clarke. "Social Organization and Risk." In *Organizations, Uncertainty, and Risk,* pp. 309–21. Boulder: Westview Press, 1992.

———, eds. *Organizations, Uncertainty, and Risk.* Boulder: Westview Press, 1992.

Shryock, Richard H. "The History of Quantification in Medical Science." *Isis* 52, part 2 (June 1961): 215–37.

Sills, David L. *The Volunteers: Means and Ends in a National Organization.* Glencoe, Ill.: Free Press, 1957.

Smith, Bruce L. R. *The Advisors: Scientists and the Policy Process.* Washington D.C.: Brookings Institution, 1992.

Smith, Jane S. *Patenting the Sun: Polio and the Salk Vaccine.* New York: Doubleday, 1990.

———. "Suspended Judgement: Remembering the Role of Thomas Francis, Jr., in the Design of the 1954 Salk Vaccine Trial." *Controlled Clinical Trials* 13 (1992): 181–84.

Star, Susan Leigh. "Scientific Work and Uncertainty." *Social Studies of Science* 15 (1985): 391–427.

Starr, Chauncey. "Social Benefit versus Technological Risk." *Science* 165 (September 19, 1969): 1232–38.

Starr, Paul. *The Social Transformation of American Medicine.* New York: Basic Books, 1982.

Stehr, Nico. "The Ethos of Science Revisited: Social and Cognitive Norms." *Sociological Inquiry* 48 (1978): 172–96.

Steinbrook, Robert. "Protecting Research Subjects: The Crisis at Johns Hopkins." *New England Journal of Medicine* 346, no. 9 (2002): 716–20.

Stevens, M. L. Tina. *Bioethics in America: Origins and Cultural Politics.* Baltimore: Johns Hopkins University Press, 2000.

Stewart, Irvin. *Organizing Scientific Research for War.* Boston: Little, Brown, 1948.

Stewart, Larry R. *The Rise of Public Science: Rhetoric, Technology, and Natural Philosophy in Newtonian Britain, 1660–1750.* Cambridge: Cambridge University Press, 1992.

Stinchcombe, Arthur L. *Information and Organizations.* Berkeley and Los Angeles: University of California Press, 1990.

Stone, Deborah A. "The Resistible Rise of Preventive Medicine" In *Health Policy in Transition,* ed. Lawrence D. Brown, pp. 103–28. Durham: Duke University Press, 1987.

Suchman, Mark C., and Lauren B. Edelman. "Legal Rational Myth: The New Institutionalism and the Law and Society Tradition." *Law and Social Inquiry* 21, no. 4 (fall 1996): 903–41.

Sutton, John R., and Frank Dobbin. "The Two Faces of Governance: Responses to Legal Uncertainty in U.S. Firms, 1955 to 1985." *American Sociological Review* 61 (1996): 794–811.

Swazey, Judith, and Renée C. Fox. "The Clinical Moratorium: A Case Study of Mitral Valve Surgery." In *Experimentation with Human Subjects,* ed. Paul A. Freund, pp. 315–57. New York: George Braziller, 1970.

Swidler, Ann. "Culture in Action: Symbols and Strategies." *American Sociological Review* 51 (1986): 273–86.

Tomes, Nancy. *The Gospel of Germs: Men, Women, and the Microbe in American Life.* Cambridge: Harvard University Press, 1998.

Toumey, Christopher P. *Conjuring Science: Scientific Symbols and Cultural Meanings in American Life.* New Brunswick: Rutgers University Press, 1996.

Tröhler, Urich. "Human Research: From Ethos to Law, from National to International Regulation." In *Historical and Philosophical Perspectives on Biomedical Ethics: From Paternalism to Autonomy?* ed. Andreas-Holger Maehle and Johanna Geyer-Kordesch, pp. 95–118. Aldershot, England: Ashgate, 2002.

———. *To Improve the Evidence of Medicine: The Eighteenth Century British Origins of a Critical Approach.* Edinburgh: College of Physicians of Edinburgh, 2000.

Tröhler, Ulrich, and Stella Reiter-Theil, eds. *Ethical Codes in Medicine: Foundations and Achievements of Codification since 1947.* Aldershot, England: Ashgate, 1998.

Turner, Barry A. "The Organizational and Interorganizational Development of Disasters." *Administrative Science Quarterly* 21 (1976): 378–97.

Vaughan, Diane. *The Challenger Launch Decision.* Chicago: University of Chicago Press, 1996.

———. "Regulating Risk: Implications of the Challenger Accident." In *Organizations, Uncertainties, and Risk,* ed. James F. Short and Lee Clarke, pp. 235–53. Boulder: Westview Press, 1992.

Warner, John Harley. *The Therapeutic Perspective: Medical Practice, Knowledge, and Identity in America, 1820–1885.* Cambridge: Harvard University Press, 1986.

Weber, Max. *Economy and Society: An Interpretive Sociology.* 1924. Ed. Guenther Roth and Claus Wittich. 2 vols. Berkeley and Los Angeles: University of California Press, 1978.

White, G. Edward. *Tort Law in America: An Intellectual History.* New York: Oxford University Press, 1980.

Wilson, Daniel J. "A Crippling Fear: Experiencing Polio in the Era of FDR." *Bulletin of the History of Medicine* 72 (1998): 464–95.

Wilson, Graham S. *The Hazards of Immunization.* London: Athlone Press, 1967.

Wilson, John Rowan. *Margin of Safety.* New York: Doubleday, 1963.

Wolpe, Paul Root. "The Triumph of Autonomy in American Bioethics: A Sociological Perspective." In *Bioethics and Society: Constructing the Ethical Enterprise,* ed. Raymond DeVries and Janardan Subedi, pp. 38–59. Upper Saddle River, N.J.: Prentice-Hall, 1998.

Woodward, Theodore D. *The Armed Forces Epidemiology Board.* Falls Church, Va.: Office of the Surgeon General, Department of the Army, 1990.

Zuckerman, Harriet. "Deviant Behavior and Social Control in Science." In *Deviance and Social Change,* ed. Edward Sagarin, pp. 87–138. Beverly Hills: Sage, 1977.

Zussman, Robert. "Sociological Perspectives on Medical Ethics and Decision-Making." *Annual Review of Sociology* 23 (1997): 171–89.

Zussman, Robert. *Intensive Care: Medical Ethics and the Medical Profession.* Chicago: University of Chicago Press, 1992.

Index

Recombinant DNA Advisory Committee (RAC) (*continued*) cerns regarding OTC protocol, 141–42, 205n.8; Human Gene Therapy Subcommittee, 140; purview scaled back, 142, 143; Wilson's influence with, 142, 205n.12

Reed, Walter (yellow fever experiment), 96, 192n.15

regulation: of biologicals (NIH), 50, 54, 58–59, 63, 177n.69; consumer-product safety standards, 202n.18; of experimental medical products (FDA), 1, 118, 131; federal human-subjects codes (DHHS), 118, 121–22; regulatory regimes, 202n.17; of technological hazards, 127–28, 202n.17, 203n.18. *See also* Food and Drug Administration; National Institutes of Health (NIH), 1930–44; Recombinant DNA Advisory Committee; research oversight; technological hazards

research abuses, 118–19, 120–21

research accidents: Gelsinger's death, 133, 135, 149; Roche's death, 133, 136, 138. *See also* vaccine injuries

research community (medical): capacity for moral oversight, 124–25; colleague exchanges, 14, 43, 46, 109; concern with public sentiment about risk, 113–14, 200n.74; efforts to shape public perceptions of risk, 125–27; relations with medical practitioners, 13–14; response to antivivisectionism, 32–33, 34–36, 98, 111–112, 199n.65; visibility of internal conflict, 129, 203n.22. *See also* gift culture of science; problem groups; research network (poliovirus); science (medical)

research network (gene therapy): question human use of OTC vector, 140–41, 205nn. 9–11; pursue venture capital arrangements, 152, 207n.34, 208n.35. *See also* gene therapy; gift culture of science; problems groups; research community

research network (poliovirus): capacity for moral oversight, 42–43, 64–65; change in power dynamics, 51; colleague exchanges, 43, 46; concern with public

trust, 42, 61–63, 64–65, 169n.4; Flexner's role in, 46, 51; numbers of scientists, 43, 170n.5; observe informal morality, 45–47, 52; stop vaccine use, 41–42

research oversight, stages in, 117–18. *See also* Food and Drug Administration; institutional review boards; organizational sponsors; problem groups; Recombinant DNA Advisory Committee; regulation; research community; research network (poliovirus); scientific advisory panels; social control

Richards, Alfred N., 100, 103

risk: acceptability of linked to cultural climate, 115, 200n.76; access to information about, impeded by FDA, 144; assessment of, and institutional review boards, 138–39, 140, 151; consent and, 91, 92, 95–96; disclosure of, and venture capital firms, 153; divergent stances toward, 68, 70–71t, 79–80; efforts to shape perceptions of, 111–15, 125–27, 201n.77; field of risk analysis, 200n.75; knowledgeability about, 81–83; need for expert assessment of, 132, 138, 144–45, 150–51; need for open access to information about, 153; perceptions of in lesser-harm logic, 24–25, 163n.19; procedures for managing, 91, 92, 95, 100–107; public sentiment about, 113–15, 200n.74; risk-benefits arguments, 39; strategies for managing, 88–99, 190nn. 72–73; voluntary vs. involuntary, 97. *See also* legal liability for injuries; technological hazards; vaccine injuries

River, Thomas, 52, 55; on Brodie's vaccine, 53, 56, 58, 60; on Kolmer's vaccine, 56, 58; on Leake's confrontation with Kolmer, 59, 63; and Vaccine Advisory Committee's instructions to Sabin, 79

Roche, Ellen, 133, 136

Rockefeller Foundation (International Health Division), 44; funds Kramer, 72; funds Park and Brodie, 48, 69; funds Stokes, 75; knowledgeability about risk, 81t, 82; lacks disincentives for assuming risk, 84; leaves decisions about risks to Kramer, 72; leaves decisions about risks

MORALITY AND SOCIETY SERIES

Edited by Alan Wolfe